K. Draenert · Y. Draenert · U. Garde · Ch. Ulrich, Manual of Cementing Technique

Springer
Berlin
Heidelberg
New York
Barcelona
Hong Kong
London
Milan
Paris
Singapore
Tokyo

K. Draenert · Y. Draenert · U. Garde · Ch. Ulrich

Manual of Cementing Technique

In Collaboration with
K. Blaesius, Stolberg; M. Börner, Frankfurt; K. E. Brinkmann, Karlsbad-Langensteinbach; H. Eckhardt, Vogtareuth; J. Eulert, Würzburg; B. Gerber, Neuchâtel; M. Haas, Rome; H. G. Hermichen, Neuss; D. Hohmann, Erlangen; M. Immenkamp, Markgröningen; E. König, Würzburg; R. Labitzke, Schwerte; D. Mack, Tegernsee; F. D. Malcher, Bad Winsheim; J. R. Neff, Omaha; F. Niethard, Aachen; J. Older, Midhurst; W. J. Radke, Munich; B. Rischke, Pinneberg; W. Siebert, Kassel; T.J.J.H. Slooff, Westerbeek; H. W. Springorum, Bad Mergentheim; L. Tessari, Milan; N. Walker, Markgröningen; L. Wolf, Bonn

With 153 Figures in 178 Parts

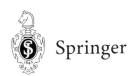

Prof. Dr. K. Draenert
Zentrum für Orthopädische Wissenschaften
Gabriel-Max-Str. 3
D–81545 München

Dr. Y. Draenert
Zentrum für Orthopädische Wissenschaften
Gabriel-Max-Str. 3
D–81545 München

Dr. U. Garde
St.-Elisabeth-Hospital
Chirurgische Abteilung
D–58638 Iserlohn

Prof. Dr. Ch. Ulrich
Klinik am Eichert
Unfallchirurgische Klinik
Postfach 660
D–73006 Göppingen

ISBN 3-450-65437-2 Springer-Verlag Berlin Heidelberg New York
Cataloging-in-Publication Data applied for

Die Deutsche Bibliothek – CIP-Einheitsaufnahme
Manual of cementing technique / by K. Draenert ... – Berlin ; Heidelberg ; New York ;
Barcelona ; Hongkong ; London ; Mailand ; Paris ; Singapur ; Tokyo ; Springer 1999
ISBN 3-540-65437-2

This work is subject to copyright. All rights are reserved, whether the whole or part of the material is concerned, specifically the rights of translation, reprinting, reuse of illustrations, recitation, broadcasting, reproduction on microfilm or in any other way, and storage in data banks. Duplication of this publication or parts thereof is permitted only under the provisions of the German Copyright Law of September 9, 1965, in its current version, and permission for use must always be obtained from Springer-Verlag. Violations are liable for prosecution under the German Copyright Law.

© Springer-Verlag Berlin Heidelberg 1999
Printed in Germany

The use of general descriptive names, registered names, trademarks, etc. in this publication does not imply, even in the absence of a specific statement, that such names are exemt from the relevant protective laws and regulations and therefore free for general use.
Product liability: The publishers cannot guarantee the accuracy of any information about the application of operative techniques and medications contained in this book. In every individual case the user must check such information by consulting the relevant literature.

Cover design: E. Kirchner, D-69121 Heidelberg
Typesetting: FotoSatz Pfeifer GmbH, D-82166 Gräfelfing
SPIN: 10555023   24/3135 – 5 4 3 2 1 0 – Printed on acid-free paper

A Tribute to Sir John Charnley

> A very important piece of work in my Unit has been the development of cold curing acrylic cement. This fundamental technique has completely revolutionised hip joint surgery.
> Charnley 1964

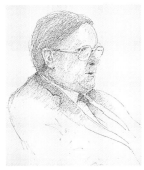

A sketch of Sir John Charnley by his son Tristram (kindly provided by T.J.J.H. Slooff)

The use of bone cement was an integral part of Charnley's low-friction arthroplasty. He was not the first person to use acrylic cement in orthopaedic surgery. Kiaer and Jansen of Copenhagen had attached plastic cups to the femoral head with acrylic cement, and reported this to an International Orthopaedic Meeting in 1951, which Charnley attended. Two years later Haboush of New York published an article in the *Bulletin of the Hospital of Joint Diseases* which indicated that he had used acrylic cement as seating compound to distribute load from a femoral prosthesis with a long stem over the bone of the femoral neck. These were failures, the result of using too little cement in the wrong place.

Charnley's meticulous studies of acrylic cement were of great importance in demonstrating the manner in which fixation was obtained and the interpretation of the long-term changes in the neighbouring tissues. Smith, a chemist and then lecturer in the Department of Material Sciences at the Turner Dental Hospital, Manchester, remembers that in 1956 Charnley asked whether he knew of a suitable material to fix a prosthesis inside the femur. Self-curing acrylic cement – polymethylmethacrylate – was used. Charnley experimented in the laboratory using a plastic femur mounted in a box – his "stuffing" box. After investigation and rehearsal outside the body, he performed his first operation with cement in Manchester 1958.

Charnley reported his first six cases in the *British Journal of Bone and Joint Surgery* in 1960. He emphasised that the dough should be "rammed" deeply into the femur by thumb pressure. The cement acted as a "grout" and not a "glue". Fixation was by interlocking and not by adhesion. The cement was forced into every crevice in the interior of the femur so that the weight of the body was dispersed over a large area of bone. The way was now clear for the introduction of cement into the hip replacement operations which Charnley was developing: first to fix the femoral prosthesis and later the socket.

Charnley continued to observe and study the effects of cement; clinical, radiological and histological in both his original group and later patients. The culmination of this stage of his research was the publication of his book *Acrylic Cement in Orthopaedic Surgery* in 1970. In this book Charnley made some interesting comments on "elasticity in the cement bond". He suggested that if one considers the transmission of load from a rough cement surface to a cancellous structure, the latter can be regarded as a system of springs. The superficial layer of cancellous bone in contact with the surface of the cement will "move as one" with the cement surface when load is applied. The deflection of the cancellous structure under load takes place inside the bulk of the cancellous bone. In this way he maintained that we can explain the paradox of the transmission of load from a hard to a soft substance without relative motion taking place between the surfaces in contact. Charnley wrote "it is on these grounds that I believe it is an advantage to have a layer of cancellous bone interposed between a cement surface and the cortical bone".

Failure of early attempts to use acrylic cement in orthopaedic surgery was the result of surgeons having an incorrect mental picture of the way in which cement functions. It is not an adhesive "glue", nor should it be used merely as an adjunct to mechanical fixation. Charnley considered his contribution to this subject was the concept of achieving fixation entirely by means of cement. He believed the most important zone for the cement was between the distal two-thirds of the stem of the femoral implant and the strong tubular shaft of the cortical bone. He distrusted the cancellous bone of the trochanters for weight bearing and sought to by-pass this region to reach sound tubular bone. In the preparation of the medullary canal of the femur, Charnley did not advise curettage of the cancellous lining, for he maintained that the cancellous layer contributes to firm anchorage and may contribute some slight elasticity to counter the abrupt change in Young's modulus between bone of the cortex and the cement. Charnley reasoned that cancellous bone is important for anchorage of cement but mistrusted it for load bearing – a concept from his studies on bone healing in 1961.

Throughout his work, one thought was always dominant in Charnley's mind: the best time to use acrylic cement is the first time, when the gritty surface of fresh cancellous bone can best accept cement. Painstaking attention to detail was mandatory to avoid mechanical failure and build for 20 years, not just the next year or two. Acrylic cement is widely used in many different parts of the world. Complications arise from inadequate technical skills by operators. Implant failure seriously threatens the reputation of cement and will hold back the process of science.

When Charnley described the procedure for the low-friction arthroplasty, he suggested it should be seen as an exercise in practical mechanical engineering – not a surgical operation. The technique is broken down into a sequence of precise steps, each of which can be illustrated and facilitated by a special tool.

It was imperative to Charnley to obtain post-mortem material from highly successful cases. By 1982 there were 78 specimens of hip prosthesis. Before he could investigate this unique collection, Charnley died. The project was undertaken by Malcolm, who showed "a beautiful bone interlock between viable bone and cement" around the femoral prosthesis.

Klaus and Yvette Draenert tread in the path laid by Charnley, and as with him, they performed painstaking, meticulous, scientific experiments on the use of cement and its morphological and histological relationship with the bone and implants. Their unique contribution has been to emphasise the dynamic importance of the interface between implant and bone in both the cemented and uncemented prosthesis. This three-dimensional reconstruction of the interface has been a land mark in understanding the morphology and histology which contributes to the fixation and longevity of implants. They have shown that cement transmits energy to spongiosa bone which is then strengthened. The results have affected the technical details of the operation leading to a stepwise procedure in mechanical engineering to improve the use of bone cement. Thus cancellous bone is stiffened by bone cement to carry the load and provide the patient with many years of trouble free activity.

John Charnley is admired for his meticulous evaluation of outcome – if merited it could lead to a change of mind. Sir John would have been delighted with the Draenerts' work, an extension of his own pioneering accomplishments done in the same meticulous manner. They have confirmed and enlarged on his original findings. More important, they have expanded, passing from static anchorage, across the interface, showing the dynamic concept of bone becoming stiff and strong.

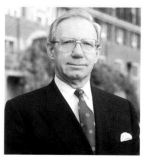

J. Older

John Older, MB BS BDS FRCS
Consultant Orthopaedic Surgeon
Royal Surrey County Hospital, Guildford, Surrey
King Edward VII Hospital, West Sussex
Honorary Senior Research Fellow, University of Surrey
United Kingdom

Foreword

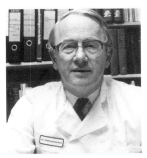

T.J.J.H. Slooff

This extensive and well-prepared manual is the work product of Klaus and Yvette Draenert, who are deeply interested in cemented total hip arthroplasty and in particular, intensely involved in related research for the past 25 years. Their damage analysis is aimed at cement fixation with the purpose to rule out any risk for the patient. They introduce the theme with a wide review of the literature on the successes and failures of the various types of total hip components. Because of the lack of standardization of the various parameters used in these studies, they do not recommend any one special type, and on the basis of this literature study they wonder why there is such a search for new types and (fixation) methods of total hip arthroplasties.

Instead of these long-term follow-up studies, the authors plead to carry out systematic histological research on retrieved human material as was firstly started and recommended by the late Sir John Charnley. Their investigations demonstrate that polymethylmethacrylate behaves biologically as an inert material that can be integrated into the bone, without a fibrous membrane interface. This could also be assessed in their animal experiments when the appropriate biomechanical conditions are provided. To achieve a connective tissue free bone-cement junction it is important to prevent deformation in the bone structures and micromotion between the bone-cement interface. The most important measure to prevent these phenomena is to stiffen the spongiosa structures with bone cement. In contrast with Charnley's cementing technique, the Draenerts recommend not removing the spongiosa but preserving and treating the spongiosa carefully, and then stiffening it. In this way the cancellous bone can carry the load!

In the past 20 years many research projects have been performed in their Scientific Centre in Munich and Berne, with practical applications in symposia, workshops and hands-on activities. Based on the results of their meticulous investigations and assisted by well-trained scientists, they have developed step by step an implantation (vacuum) technique for bone cement and implants to guarantee a safe and long-lasting clinical result. This technique encompasses in essence: choosing the right location to enter the proximal femur, the indispensable use of precision instrumentation in order not to damage the cancellous bone, the effective use of a drainage system to prevent venous emboli, and the adequate use of a lavage system with an anticoagulation solution. The cement is used in a standard viscosity state, mixed in vacuum, precompressed, and then under complete vacuum pressure suctioned into the blood free spongiosa of the acetabulum and the femur.

This manual, which is inspired by a great devotion, seeks to present and clarify a newly developed technique for cement preparation and insertion. I believe that the philosophy on which the Draenerts' method is based is realistic and scientifically well devised. It is a genuine step forward in cemented total hip arthroplasty. Although the practically and scientifically supervised results show a high reproducibility, a short surgical time, and a complication free operative procedure, we will look forward to the clinical and radiological results in the long-term.

With this manual, the authors have addressed an important issue in cemented total hip arthroplasty. They have designed their research programs in their typical manner of modesty, perseverance, honesty, and precision. These have been carried out with the continuous help and support of their team of experts and many friends from all over the world. Their message is very clear: the key to the problem in total hip arthroplasty is research of retrieved material. Very convincingly, they have given us the tools and shown us the ways to achieve adequate fixation of the components. I sincerely hope that their masterwork will be of benefit to everyone involved with the expanding orthopedic field.

T.J.J.H. Slooff, MD, Ph.D.
Professor Emeritus in Orthopaedic Surgery
at the University of Nijmegen
Westerbeek, The Netherlands
October 1998

Preface

Damage analysis is a well-known and established learning process which indicates why an object failed, such as when "human error" is to blame. Considerably rarer, even uncommon, is the analysis of success. One assumes the principles of the construction were correct until eventually damage occurs, which then sets off the damage analysis.

Did Charnley really know why his operative procedure was so successful? The surface enlargement of the anchorage is certainly one of the reasons, but this may not be the essential one. We do not know. A number of things seem to indicate the opposite, for example, his opinion of spongious bone: "Cancellous bone has in fact a very restricted form of osteogenic activity" (Charnley 1961b).

The analysis of successfully implanted prostheses according to Charnley's procedure was a very stony research project which resulted in many small findings. This knowledge, assembled as a mosaic, provided new germs of crystallization for applied research programs. Overall, the study group at the Zentrum für Orthopädische Wissenschaften in Munich have been working on the bone-to-cement interface since 1974, and reports on more than 100 research programs specifically about or relating to bone cement have now been at least in part published.

The validation procedure of all small steps involved in the Charnley technique up to the equipment of the operating theater made these studies necessary. The most important milestones in this path form the focus of this study. These research programs are presented in a comprehensive manner. The objective was to make the procedure almost perfectly reproducible, ruling out any risks for the patient.

K. Draenert, MD, PhD
Zentrum für Orthopädische Wissenschaften
Munich, Germany

Contents

1	**Historical Background**	1
1.1	Conditions Before Charnley	2
1.2	John Charnley	3
2	**Histomorphology of the Bone-to-Cement Contact**	4
2.1	The Cemented Total Hip Arthroplasty	4
2.2	Histomorphology of the Bone-to-Cement Contact (Animal Experiments)	7
2.2.1	Changes Around Normal Bone Cements	7
2.2.2	TCP/HA Bone Cements	11
2.3	Histomorphology of Human Samples	14
2.3.1	Material and Methods	14
2.3.2	Summary of Results	14
3	**Can Cancellous Bone Carry the Load?**	19
3.1	About the Deformation Behavior of Spongiosa	19
3.1.1	Elasticity	19
3.1.2	Viscoelasticity	20
3.1.3	Isotropic Deformation	20
3.1.4	Resilience and Damping	20
3.1.5	Damping	21
3.1.6	Breaking (Tensile) Strength and Toughness	21
3.1.7	Compliance	22
3.1.8	Energy	22
3.1.9	Impact	22
3.2	Deformation of Bone Through Different Implants	22
3.3	Stiffening of Spongiosa with Bone Cement	26
3.3.1	Human Histopathological Key Findings	26
3.3.2	Histomorphological Findings in the Proximal Femur After Joint Surface Replacement	28
3.3.3	Histomorphological Findings on Cancellous Bone Stiffened with Bone Cement in the Distal Epiphysis of the Femur in Rabbits	30
4	**Approach to the Hip Joint**	34
4.1	Posterolateral Approach	34
4.2	Transgluteal Approach	36
5	**Preparation of the Acetabulum**	38
5.1	Preparatory Steps	39
5.2	Exposure of the Acetabulum	39
5.3	Fossa Acetabuli	40
5.4	Preparation of the Bony Acetabulum	40
5.5	Anatomical Composition of the Joint Surface of the Acetabulum	41
5.6	Lavage, Anticoagulation and Stiffening of the Acetabular Roof	41

5.7	Inclination and Alignment	42
6	**Preparation of the Bone Cement**	**45**
6.1	Advantages of Standard Viscosity Bone Cement	45
6.2	Cold Storage as a Simple Method To Achieve a Temporarily Lower Viscosity	46
6.3	Homogeneous and Bubble-Free Mixture	47
6.4	Prepressurizing Bone Cements, a *Conditio Sine Qua Non*	50
6.5	Application of the Bubble-Free Bone Cement	53
7	**Preparation of the Femur**	**55**
7.1	Opening of the Medullary Canal and Implantation Axis	55
7.2	Surgical Diamond Instrumentation	57
7.3	Drainage of the Medullary Canal	61
7.4	Preparation of the Implant's Bed	65
7.5	Lavage	67
7.6	Plugging the Medullary Cavity	68
7.7	Heparinization, Cementation, and Implantation	70
8	**Scientific Background of Vacuum Application**	**72**
8.1	The Problem of Thromboembolism and Drainage of the Medullary Canal	72
8.2	The Distal Drill Hole	76
8.3	The Stem-Canal Volume Relationship	78
9	**Consideration of the Prosthetic Design of the Femoral Stem**	**79**
9.1	Stiffening Spongiosa of the Femur	79
9.2	Calcar Femoris	81
9.3	Stem Design	83
9.4	Preoperative Planning	86
9.4.1	Plane of the Metaphyseal "V"	86
9.4.2	Offset and Alignment	86
9.5	Centralizing Anatomical Design	92
10	**Instrumentation**	**93**
11	**Conclusions: The Success of Cemented Components**	**96**
11.1	First-Generation Cementing Techniques	96
11.2	Success of the Cemented Component Is Due to Stiffened Bone Structures	97
11.3	Cancellous Bone Stiffened by Bone Cement Can Survive	97
11.4	Preservation of Cancellous Bone	98
References		**99**
Subject Index		**107**
Author Index		**109**

CHAPTER 1

Historical Background

In the history of medicine strange and unrepeatable experiments on human beings and animals take place. Many spectacular surgical interventions were tried in a state of emergency, for example in war. Von Langenbeck (1810–1887) was one of the greatest war surgeons, and therefore one of the most creative surgical inventors that Germany knows. However, it is not only the state of emergency which leads to creativity. Bernhard Heine (1800–1846), for example, represents the restless scientist. He performed basic research, mainly with dogs, on fracture and defect healing (Heine 1836). Themistokles Gluck (Fig. 1) was rooted in the spirit of these people.

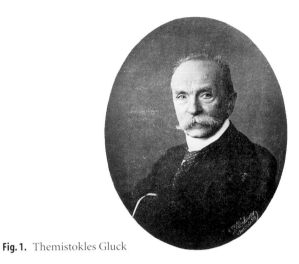

Fig. 1. Themistokles Gluck

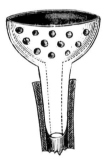

Fig. 2. Ivory piece for arthroplasty of the knee designed by Themistokles Gluck in 1890

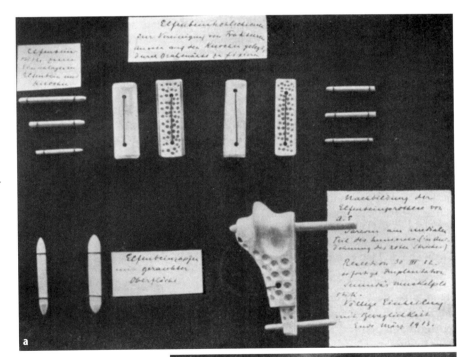

Fig. 3. Artificial ivory joint of the elbow and ivory jaw piece by König

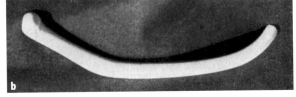

He was creative and innovative in all areas of surgery (Gluck 1891). The first joint replacement, a knee joint of ivory, was carried out by him in 1890 (Fig. 2). König implanted ivory prostheses in the upper arm and the lower jaw and could report good healings (Fig. 3; König 1913). Joint function was also tried to be repaired by producing a pseudarthrosis (Barton 1827) or by interposition of different materials into the articular space (reported in Haboush 1953). These early individual attempts to restore lost joint function form the basis for the successful quest for functional joint replacements in the 20th century.

1.1
Conditions Before Charnley

Restoring joint function by implants was certainly impeded by the lack of materials for implantation. Significant advances in metallurgy and the advent of plastics spurred a number of innovative approaches to improve joint function, particularly of the hip. Starting in 1923, Smith-Petersen (1948) worked on his idea to interpose a freely movable "mold" between the femoral head and the acetabulum to stimulate the natural repair of the degenerated cartilage. Initially he used glass for his molds but in 1938 he switched to Vitallium, a corrosion-free Co-Cr-Mo alloy. The Vitallium-mold arthroplasty was still in use in the 1950s, when Aufranc (1957) reported on more than 1000 patients treated. A different path was taken by the Judet brothers (1950) who designed a true prosthesis in the mid-1940s which replaced the degenerated part of the femoral head. Their early cup-prostheses were made entirely from polymethylmethacrylate, but disappointed and failed the practical test. However, the failure gave important lessons to the mechanical requirements for artificial joint components (Ruckelshausen 1964). The Judet-prosthesis suffered from intense wear which lead to an aggressive granuloma and disintegration of the artificial femoral head. Also, the short polymethylmethacrylate stem frequently broke which led to the use of steel in later models. Furthermore, anchorage in the bone was not stable and caused necrosis of the femoral cortex (Charnley 1961a; Anderson et al. 1964; Ruckelshausen 1964).

The next step was not merely to replace the deteriorated joint surface on the femoral head, as with the cup-prosthesis, but to completely substitute the femoral neck and head. These kinds of prostheses required the permanent removal of the femoral head and neck. They were anchored by a stem in the medullary cavity of the femur. Different models were developed in the 1950s, for example, by Haboush (1953), Thompson (1954), and Moore (1957). All were made from corrosion-resistant iron-free Co-Cr with head diameters sized to fit the unoperated acetabular joint surface. Such femoral prostheses were designed to be implanted without bone cement.

Femoral prostheses had one major disadvantage: they exerted unphysiological stress to the acetabular joint surface, yielding to unpredictable results in the long-term (Charnley 1961a; Salvati and Wilson 1973). A solution to this inevitable problem when only one component of a joint is replaced seemed to be replacing both the femoral head and the acetabular joint surface by arthroplasties. First total prostheses with a metal-metal combination were presented by Haboush in 1953. Other total hip joint implants were performed by McKee and Watson-Farrar (1966) in the 1950s. One major problem was the stable anchorage of the acetabular cup to the pelvic bone, but also of the femoral component to the femur. A possible solution put forward by Haboush (1953) was to use polymethylmethacrylate as a bone cement. Polymethylmethacrylate was invented in 1928

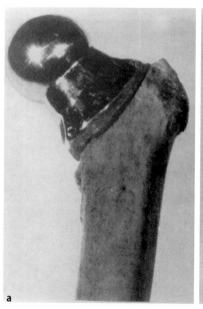 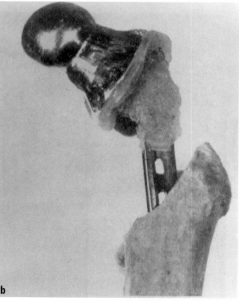

Fig. 4a,b. Femoral prostheses with intramedullary stem by Haboush (1953). **b** The prosthesis is shown partly withdrawn, documenting the proximal anchorage with bone cement

in Germany and patented as "Plexiglas." Its potential for orthopedic medicine was realized shortly thereafter. First it was applied in dentistry and to fix defects in the skullbone (Kleinschmidt 1941; Brown 1947).

Its usefulness for anchoring implants, femoral cup prostheses and also acetabular cups, was described by Kiaer (1953) and Haboush (1953; Fig. 4). It was also used as prosthesis material (Judet and Judet 1950); however, it was soon abandoned as unsuitable for that latter purpose.

1.2
John Charnley

The stage was set when Charnley entered the arena. Although significant advances had been made in developing hip joint replacements, however, not a single procedure was without significant problems. There was no doubt that hip joint replacements were still to a large extent experimental gambles. A nice monograph could be written on the history of total joint arthroplasty that would end with Charnley (1960, 1961a,b, 1964, 1970a,b,c, 1979). Precisely why did Charnley make the breakthrough?

Charnley was named the founder of artificial joint replacement because he established the first laboratory for applied surgical research, a laboratory in which the problems and questions of joint replacement were evaluated. He was certainly not aware of what a revolution he would trigger when he installed the first instruments for friction experiments in his garage. He carefully considered mechanics, biomechanics, and pathology; all in addition to his hospital activity. Thus Charnley became the father of countless research institutes and laboratories around the world.

The common denominator of all these successes was continuous, systematic, basic and applied research. One of the outstanding fellows of John Charnley in consistently passing all ideas through the experimental laboratory in a very efficient and systematic way is Tom Slooff from Nijmegen. He performed classical studies on the bone-to-cement issue (Slooff 1971, 1972). Charnley had many loyal successors conducting clinical and research work from whom Mike Wroblewsky (1986, 1990, 1993) in Wrightington, John Older (1986, 1995) in Midhurst, and Edouardo Salvati (Salvati and Wilson 1973; Salvati et al. 1976, 1981) and Nas Eftekhar (Eftekhar 1971, 1987; Eftekhar and Tzitzikalakis 1986) in New York represent these outstanding personalities who continue to put forward the ingenious spirit of Sir John.

Charnley's operative procedure is still the most successful. His combination of a solid intramedullary anchorage of the femoral prosthesis and also of the acetabular cup with bone cement, the design of a femoral prosthesis with a low-friction 22-mm diameter head, and the use of a metal/plastic (first Teflon, later polyethylene) joint interface lead to the breakthrough. Charnley was not able to finish his work, however, and many questions concerning the reproducibility and tolerance of his procedure were left unanswered. Minor, peripheral appearing, details remained unaddressed although they, as later turned out, had unexpected far-reaching implications, for example the cementing technique.

Certainly Charnley would have worked on all questions in detail, for no one had taken charge of the hospital cases the way he had, both in the clinic and in his laboratory. Therefore John Charnley is rightfully named the founder of artificial joint replacement. There are many ideas, but the way to the validated procedure is a stony and thorny one.

CHAPTER 2

Histomorphology of the Bone-to-Cement Contact

2.1
The Cemented Total Hip Arthroplasty

If one report contains 25-year results (Wroblewski 1993; Older 1995; Kobayashi et al. 1996) from an operative procedure, but another speaks of "cement disease" (Jones and Hungerford 1987), a more specific scientific analysis of the unreproducibility of the operative results must be undertaken. The basic findings of the studies by Charnley (Charnley 1960, 1964; Charnley and Crawford 1968; Charnley et al. 1968; Charnley 1970a,b,c, 1979) and by McKee and Watson-Farrar (1965, 1966, 1970) concerning cement anchorage of prosthesis components cannot sufficiently explain the broad mean variation of positive and negative results.

Despite the vastly different loosening rates that can be found in the literature (Table 1), the results, and especially the results, of the cemented components are amazingly good. In the list of complications by Smith and Turner (1973), a study of 3,482 cemented total hip endoprotheses, loosening does not yet play a factor (under 0.06%) in the first year. In fact, serious complications such as pulmonary embolism (1.47%), fatal death (0.11%), and an infection rate of 1.6%, the main complication at that time, exceed them.

Dall (1975) reports more than 100 Charnley surgeries with a 95% success rate over a period of 6 months to 3 years.

As early as 1975 a randomized clinical study of Charnley prostheses and cement-free Ring total hip endoprostheses was conducted (Convery et al. 1975). This took place at a time when the complication rate shot up due to severe cardiovascular incidents, as expressed in the Dall study. Out of 100 cases he mentioned 4 pulmonary emboli, of which one was deadly, and at least one other death occurred as a result of thrombosis of the iliac vein. The randomized study by Convery et al. (1975) came to the same conclusion, namely that intraoperative changes in the cardiovascular function occurred in patients who had bone cement implanted. However, the reasons for these complications could not be resolved, even though the authors managed to prove that the toxicity of the monomer was not responsible.

In the following years, medium-term results with cemented components were published. These publications are interesting for they can be consulted and compared to the modern cementing techniques.

In 1976 Salvati et al. published the results of a series of 100 Charnley prostheses. Although the authors described a "radiolucent zone" on half of the femur components, they classified only 4 of the hips, the ones that broke distally and medially, (4%) as loosened. At least 19 of 100 femurs showed radiolucent lines of 1–2 mm,

Reference	No. of operated joints	Average stability (years)	Mean variation (years)	Overall loosening rate (%)
Salvati et al. (1976)	100	3	1–7	23
Beckenbaugh and Ilstrup (1978)	255	5.9	4.1–7.6	24
Blacker and Charnley (1978)	169	9.9	7–13	17.2
Griffith et al. (1978)	547	8.3	7– 9	14.8
Stauffer (1982)	231	10	8–13	29.9
Harris and McGann (1986)	117	6.2	5–7.1	3.4
Eftekhar and Tzitzikalakis (1986)	499	–	5–15	3.6
Rusotti et al. (1988)	251	5	5–7	2.4

Table 1. Loosening rates

while in 36 femurs radiolucent lines of 1 mm or less were seen. In 3 of the 4 loosenings a transverse fracture of the distal cement border occurred. If one adds the imminent loosenings of the femoral component of 19% to the definite loosening of 4%, this amounts to 23% loosened femur components in a time range averaging 3 years. Beckenbaugh and Ilstrup (1978) published a study of 255 verified Charnley prostheses that had been implanted an average for 5.9 years (Table 1). With these prostheses they found about the same percentage (24%) of loosened femur components. From the Charnley hospital in Wrightington, Blacker and Charnley (1978) reported on 169 patients with a 7- to 13-year follow-up (9.9 years on average). Although Blacker and Charnley listed only four definite femoral component loosenings, the equivalent of 2.4%, one must take into account the grade II demarcation as an imminent loosening in order to be able to compare with the studies of Salvati et al. (1976) and Beckenbaugh and Ilstrup (1978). With this group included we now have 29 components, the equivalent of 17.2%, with the numbers not being far apart.

Griffith et al. (1978) were in the position to do 7- to 9-year follow-ups (8.3 years average) on 547 Charnley hips. Stating 2.8% definite loosenings and 12% imminent loosenings, the authors are around the loosening rate of 14.8% after an average of 8.3 years. Their stated loosening rate of 2.8% cannot be compared directly to the previous one due to the evaluation method. Overall these authors come conclusively to the same results of 14.2% mechanical loosenings.

In the 10-year follow-up of 100 patients in the publications of 1976; Salvati et al. (1981) found that only 5 of the 74 radiologically examined cases had definite loosenings and one a fracture of the shaft, which equals 11.1%. The radiolucent lines mentioned and listed in the study do not allow a relevant correlation to imminent loosenings. After all, 50% (27 out of 54 controlled X-rays) showed such zones.

Stauffer (1982) reexamined the patients who previously had been examined by Beckenbaugh and Ilstrup (1978) 10 years ago. He found 29.9% loosened femoral components on 231 hips, which indicates a flattening of the heretofore rapidly rising loosening curve.

Sutherland et al. (1982) published the first 10-year results of the Müller prosthesis with the curved shaft (banana). They found a loosening rate of 40% with this femoral component. Wroblewski (1986) published the 15- to 21-year results from Wrightington in which he states that out of 116 low-friction arthroplasties 85.3% stayed absolutely painless and 78% experienced almost complete freedom of motion in the joint.

In 1986 Röttger and Elson published the results of the Buchholz "St. Georg" prosthesis. They used survival curves in their representation and found a loosening rate of approximately 11.4% in which femoral components with a radiolucent zone under 2 mm were counted together with the solid anchored prosthesis. In other studies such femoral components would have been regarded as imminent loosenings.

John Older (1986) published a 10- to 12-year follow-up study on the original Charnley hip in which he reports only 2% aseptic loosenings of 153 artificial joints. A differentiation of the radiological findings in view of a radiolucent zone was not taken into account in this study. Likewise, Brady and McCutchen (1986) did not take into consideration exact radiological analysis in their 10-year study results of 170 Charnley prostheses, ending up with a revision rate of 8.8%. Hamilton and Joyce (1986) reported on more than 196 Charnley LFAs (Low-Friction Arthroplasties) that were from 3 to 11 years old. Due to the documented radiological findings, at least 12.6% of the cases can be considered as loosened and if the osteolytical changes are added, 17%. On the same prosthesis type (Charnley-LFA), Eftekhar and Tzitzikalakis (1986) published 5- to 15-year results of 499 primary surgeries. They found a stability of approximately 9.4 years, and a failure rate of only 2.4%, more precisely 4.5% including the imminent loosenings (Eftekhar 1987: same percentage). Terayama studied two groups: 13 LFAs greater than 10 years old had a loosening rate of 7.7%, according to described findings, and 107 LFAs more than 5 years old with a loosening rate of 1.6%, in addition to a probable loosening of another 5.8% which is all together 7.4% (Terayama 1986). The difficulty of assessing and comparing the follow-up studies can be seen in the Dall et al. (1986) study. Dall followed 88 Charnley LFAs which had been implanted for an average of 12 years; 9.2% were reported as loosened shafts (the broken ones and those described as loose) which comes to 13.3%. However, if one adds the shafts that showed a radiolucent zone under 2 mm, the total is 22.4%.

Russotti et al. (1988) checked 251 cemented arthroplasties of the Harris II type which had been cemented in the modern method, according to his publication (Harris and McGann 1986). They compared their results to previous results of studies by Beckenbaugh and Ilstrup (1978) and Stauffer (1982). Their follow-ups included 5- to 7-year-old prostheses, on average all above 5 years old, which were easy to compare with the study of Beckenbaugh and Ilstrup (1978) who at that time reported 24% loosenings. Using the same study method Russotti et al. came to 1.2% definite loosenings, 0.4% probable loosenings and 0.8% possible loosenings which all together gives a loosening rate of 2.4%. Since these studies are absolutely comparable, one can conclude, as Harris and McGann (1986) had done already, that 5–6 years after surgery the improved cementing technique had improved the results tenfold. Comparing the Beckenbaugh and Ilstrup (1978) results with the 1988 Russotti et al. results illustrates how deceptive the clinical findings of the analyses on the condition of the artificial joint can be. The Beckenbaugh study group, too, had a success rate of 85% of good and excellent results concerning the clinical subjective and objective judgment, although 24% of the femoral components had to be classified as loosened.

Even the newer studies which partly present 20-year results (Hoffman 1990) demonstrate that it is very difficult to compare individual studies with others, for the comparison parameters had not been standardized. Using the Kaplan and Meier (1958) survival curve, the newer studies of 1,163 primary total hip endoprostheses surgeries show the Charnley prosthesis was 96% successful after 5 years, 88% successful after 10 years, and 73% successful after 15 years. They are therefore more successful than the compared Müller standard prostheses. General conclusions can be made concerning the poor reproducibility of individual prostheses and operative procedures, but specific conclusions can only be drawn extremely carefully. Even studies that followed the survival curve by Kaplan and Meier (1958) do not help significantly when it comes to analyzing the reproducibility of a method, and comprehending the detailed biological process and underlying principles.

Thus the Carter et al. (1990) study, for example, only gives a very limited report concerning the anchorage stability and anchorage durability of the individual components, because one must strictly separate problems of the socket versus problems of the femoral stem anchorage. One needs to keep in mind that the Carter study, after all, covers 493 hip joints with an average durability of 12.9 years and managed to confirm a survival rate of 91% for the 10-year-, 87% for the 15-year-, and at least 82% for the 20-year prostheses. It is amazing that with such good results there is nevertheless a constant search for new methods on the artificial hip joint replacement, especially methods without the use of bone cement.

A comparison becomes impossible when a different anchorage philosophy (e.g., the Exeter HIP-system with its follow-up studies) is compared with clinical studies of more conventional prosthesis designs. The quick subsiding and setting of the prosthesis was equated with loosening, or at least the probable loosening, of the component from a conventional prosthesis. The anchorage philosophy of the Exeter HIP system is based on the cold-flow characteristic of the bone cement which gets radially pressed into the bone while the prosthesis with its high polished surface subsides into the cement sheath (Ling 1981). A conclusion of anchorage stability can only be drawn from the number of fractures of the cement sheath and the time dependent subsiding of the components (Chenet et al. 1997). Ling (1981) carried out 418 surgeries with 225 follow-ups and showed an average durability of 7.3 years. Different insertion depths of 1 mm to 10 mm could be measured. In this series 31 cement fractures could be recognized with the naked eye, so these cases should be classified as "probably loose"

which would lead to a loosening rate of 13.4%. His description of the diaphyseal hypertrophy correlated as well with the grade of subsidence, thus one can conclude that the stems with a high subsidence must be considered loose. If the limit is set at 2 mm, this would indicate 20.5% loosened stems.

Regardless of how clinical studies are evaluated, they cannot give details about what happens in the tissue of the bony bed. Therefore, a reliable analysis of these biological processes can still only be found by systematic histological research with preparations from institutes of pathology. However, research and sampling of such preparations for histological evaluation is expensive and explains why few histological studies have been conducted until now. New preparation and documentation methods became necessary in order to demonstrate an artifact-free implant-to-bone interface. In addition, an understanding of the overall reaction of the bone to the implant had to be developed. This included a thorough histological study of the bone with its different compartments of the implant anchorage so that its reaction could be evaluated. For the documentation a three-dimensional reconstruction of the histological reaction pattern around the prosthesis was established. The bone-to-cement interface could be investigated artifact-free due to new processing methods. It was shown that newly formed bone can closely contact with the polymethylmethacrylate (PMMA) implant, without connective tissue (Draenert 1981); furthermore, the bone matrix demineralizes ("changed bone"; Charnley 1979) depending on the relative motion occurring in the interface; connective tissue and giant cells, osteoclasts, and free foreign body giant cells only appeared when the relative motion in the interface exceeded a certain degree (Draenert 1981; Haddad et al. 1996; Goodman et al. 1997; Hukkanen et al. 1997; Van der Vis et al. 1998).

The correlations between the smooth surface of the bone cement, the relative motion, and the tangential orientation of the newly formed bone along the cement, directly adhering onto the cement when the surface is roughened by hydroxyapatite and tricalcium phosphate, were published (Draenert 1986).

Systematic human pathological studies were carried out only by Charnley (1970a,b,c, 1979), Draenert (1986, 1988, 1990) and Malcolm (1990). Some informative sections of up to 17.5-year-old femoral stems and X-rays of sections were published by Jasty et al. (1990). These findings confirmed the studies by Draenert (1988) in which robust bony anchorages had been demonstrated in prostheses which were worn complaint-free for many years until death. Linder and Hansson (1983) by means of a transmission electron microscope finally confirmed connective tissue-free bone-to-cement contacts on tissue samples taken during revision surgery.

It can be accepted as scientifically verified that PMMA is a biologically inert material which can be integrated into the bone, connective tissue-free, if the appropriate biomechanical conditions are given. An implant can be evaluated, however, only if the entire bony bed can be reconstructed three-dimensionally with serial sections. Therefore, in recent years methods which enable us to do so were developed.

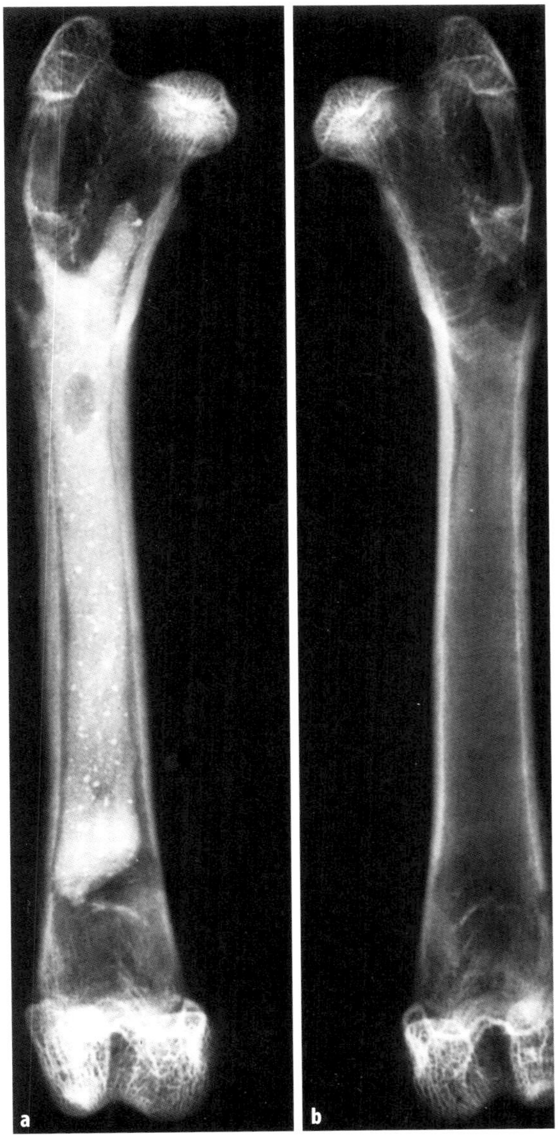

2.2 Histomorphology of the Bone-to-Cement Contact (Animal Experiments)

2.2.1 Changes Around Normal Bone Cements

The systematic changes around bone cement implants were examined in animal experiments. All together 62 giant rabbits with filling of the femoral medullary cavity (Fig. 5) were histologically evaluated (Draenert 1981). The phenomena important for the understanding of each individual step of operative procedures are therefore presented again with the key findings:

After hardening, shrinkage of the PMMA occurs and a gap forms between the bone and the bone cement: polymerization shrinkage. The bone cement shrinks towards the implant and away from the bone. This can be nicely demonstrated in a simple model (plastic syringe; Fig. 6).

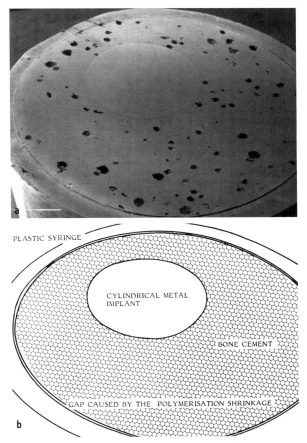

Fig. 5a,b. Experimental design of Slooff (1971): medullary canal of the femur filled with bone cement

Fig. 6a,b. Model demonstrating the shrinkage of bone cement. A plastic syringe was filled with bone cement and a metal rod was inserted; the bone cement shrank off onto the metal implant and away from the plastic, thus producing a gap

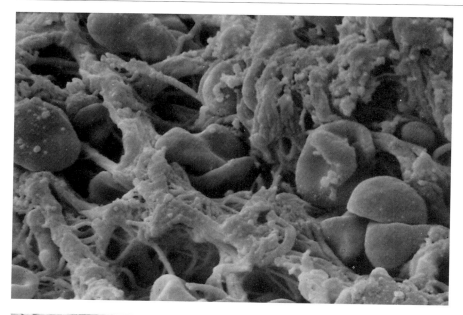

Fig. 7. Organized hematoma in the gap between cement and bone 48 h after surgery. Scanning electron microscopy (SEM)

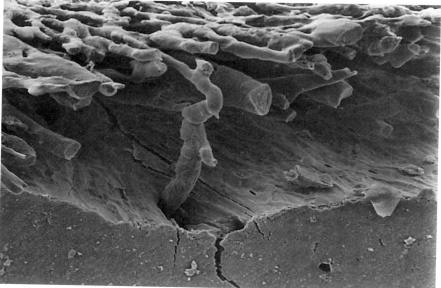

Fig. 8. A view into the gap of the interface revealing full revascularization. The bone wall is shown and two layers of delicate vessels filled with a resin; the soft tissue has been removed. A corrosion casting technique was applied. SEM 8 days after surgery

After surgery a hematoma is found in the gap between the bone and the bone cement (Fig. 7), which begins to organize itself by 48 h starting near the metaphysis.

The organization of the hematoma is followed by the revascularization (Fig. 8) and the gap healing which ends after 4 weeks. After this time the gap between the implant and the bone is compactly filled in by newly formed bone (Fig. 9), the time dependence of which is indicated by polychromatic fluorescence labeling (Fig. 10).

Depending on the completeness of the filling in of the medullary canal, periosteal bone renewal takes place with growth of a periosteal bone cuff whose thickness also depends on the stiffness of the implant (Draenert 1986; Fig. 11). Subsequent to the bone healing phase a remodeling with development of a secondary medullary cavity takes place (Fig. 12). In it we find normal bone marrow and fat cells, with marrow sinusoids and hematopoietic cell colonies.

The modeling, which is the adaptation of the bone to the implant, shows a final state after 2–3 years in animal experiments (Fig. 13): the bone cross-section is almost twice as thick, the implant in the center is supported by bone, and a normal medullary cavity has formed between the supporting structures. The same phenomenon is observed in humans after 20 years (Fig. 14).

2.2 Histomorphology of the Bone-to-Cement Contact

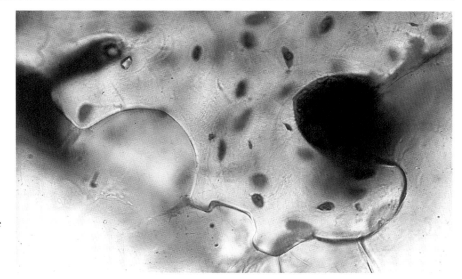

Fig. 9. Fibrous tissue-free contacts between mature lamellar bone and bone cement forming a replica of the cement's surface including a haversian vessel (*). The bone cement does not contain X-ray contrast medium

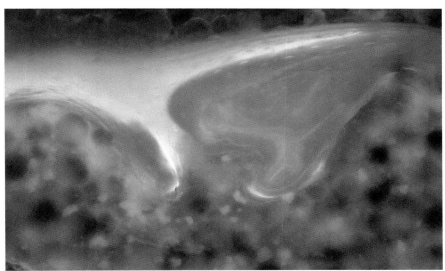

Fig. 10. Final state of the bone healing phase after 4 weeks, with demonstration of all four labels every 7 days: yellow, red, blue, and green (35-day stage). The first 5 days were not labeled, and the animal was killed 2 days after the last label

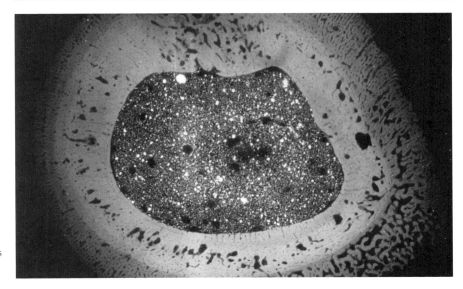

Fig. 11. The more complete the filling, the more pronounced the newly formed periosteal bone. Three weeks after surgery; microradiograph of a 60-μm section

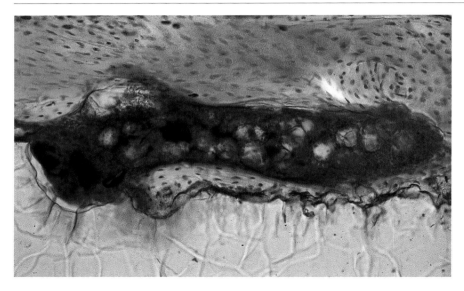

Fig. 12. The end of the bone healing process leads into the remodeling phase with reestablishment of the secondary medullary cavity, 6 months after the operation. Bone cement without contrast medium (Perspex)

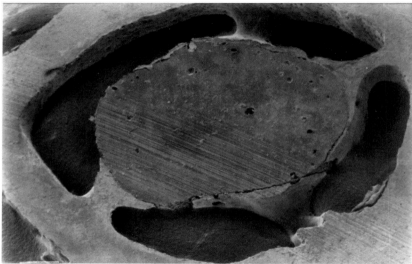

Fig. 13. The process of modeling ends after 2–2.5 years in rabbits. By this time bone has adapted to the implant, revealing the stable bony support of the implant interrupted by wide bone marrow spaces forming the secondary medullary cavity. Corroded sample

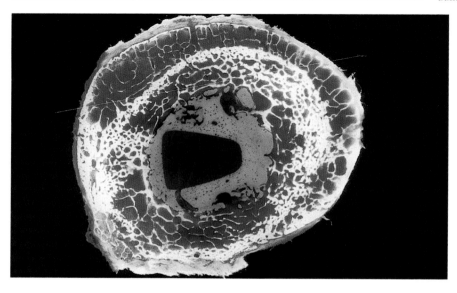

Fig. 14. The histology, 20 years after stem implantation in a human being, also shows a secondary medullary cavity with normal bone marrow. The periosteal reaction is well pronounced and contrasted to the old cortex

2.2.2
TCP/HA Bone Cements

Under favorable biomechanical conditions, a connective tissue-free bone-to-cement interface was shown in animal experiments. At the same time it was evident that a smooth surface of the PMMA bone cements was a distinct disadvantage under increasing load acting on the interface: thick osteoid layers (Linder and Hansen 1983) and tangential bone formation (Draenert 1986) showed the problem of relative motion at a smooth surface (Fig. 15). Tricalcium phosphate (TCP) and hydroxyapatite (HA) filler cements, however, did not demonstrate this problem anymore. Seventy-eight rabbits were evaluated in a histological study (Draenert 1986).

TCP/HA bone cements (Fig. 16) were superior to all other PMMA experimental attempts due to the tangential adhesion of collagen fibers onto the implant's surface.

The important advantages were: The tangential adhesion of collagen type I fibers on the implant surface. The ingrowth of the bone after reabsorption of the TCP and its associated surface enlargement (Fig. 17). The increased release of gentamicin and the replacement of the X-ray contrast medium ZrO_2 by HA. The implants were found to be bony integrated along their whole surface and supported by strong lamellar bone trabeculae (Figs. 18, 19).

The disadvantages which all filler cements show, namely a decrease in strength of the material especially in the fatigue test, were compensated by prepressurizing and vacuum-mixing.

An important side effect of all these bone cements was observed in an animal experiment with dogs in

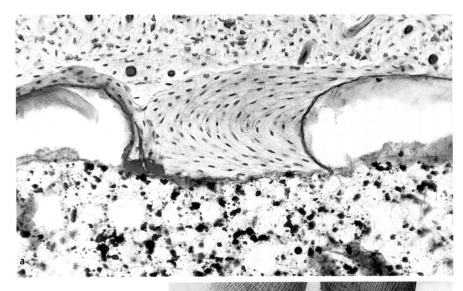

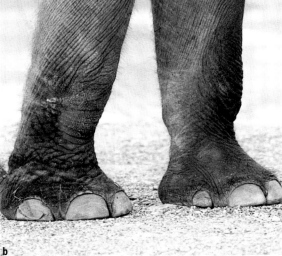

Fig. 15a,b. The supports of bone to cement are similar to an elephant foot. This formation is found on smooth but does not take place on rough surfaces. Minor surface displacements lead to demineralization, absorption, and tangential formation of connective tissue

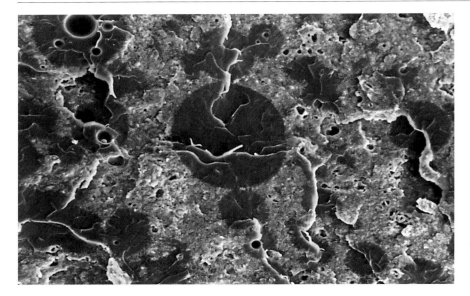

Fig. 16. The TCP/HA bone cement solves the problem of smooth surfaces of bone cements. The technical production demands porous-free filler material; otherwise monomers are soaked up by the fillers. Fractured air-dried specimen in the SEM

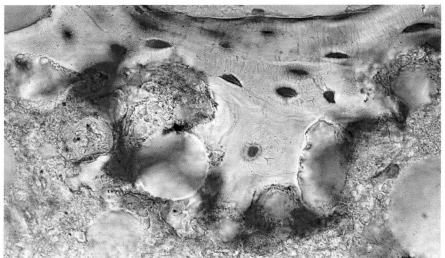

Fig. 17. The TCP bone cement is completely overgrown by bone. The absorption of filler particles is followed by a deep ingrowth into the matrix which enlarges the anchorage surface. Rabbit femur 2 years after implantation. Basic fuchsin staining

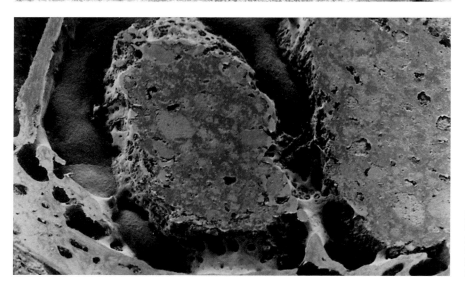

Fig. 18. The cement implant is completely covered by newly formed bone. Corroded specimen in the SEM 9 months after implantation

2.2 Histomorphology of the Bone-to-Cement Contact

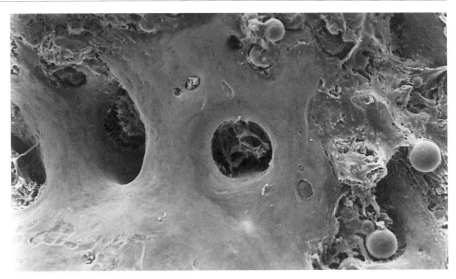

Fig. 19. Higher resolution in the SEM revealing the deep penetration by mature lamellar bone trabeculae forming a stable support

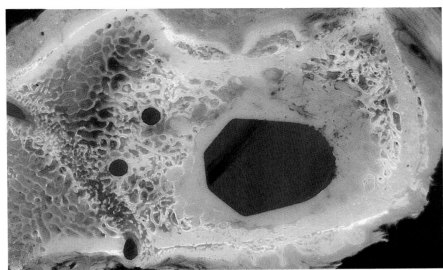

Fig. 20. Femoral component implanted into a dog's femur using the vacuum technique and the HA bone cement. The green label deep in the cement mass indicates newly formed bone, 23 days after the operation

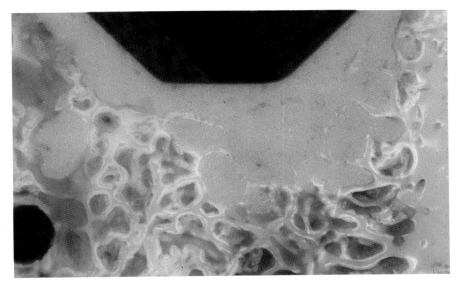

Fig. 21. Higher magnification of Fig. 20 in the HIIFL microscope, revealing newly formed bone. The yellow (8 days) and green labels (3rd week) are clearly visible

which femoral components were implanted using the vacuum application technique and HA-bone cements. A very fast revascularization took place deep into the cement mass. The polychromatic fluorescence labeling revealed newly formed bone in the gaps due to shrinkage between bone cement and bone. Twenty-three days after the operation the green label appeared deep in the cement sheath (Figs. 20, 21).

2.3
Histomorphology of Human Samples

2.3.1
Material and Methods

In the Center of Orthopedic Sciences cadaver specimens with replaced joints have been collected since 1974. These specimens came from different pathologies from around the world. In addition, samples were collected from clinics in which revisions or sometimes amputations were performed.

The specimens had been prepared through immersion-fixation in phosphate-buffered 4% formalin for months, and X-rays were taken on mammography films without image intensifying. At this moment the collection covers more than 400 cadaver specimens with replaced joints which are under investigation from different perspective views.

For the histological evaluation the preparations are first sawed in serial cross sections using a wet grinding process, and then analyzed in a plan-parallel sequence in the high intensity incident fluorescent light (HIIFL) microscope. Detail histology was taken from embedded and bloc-stained specimens using Epon 812 after having been dehydrated through graded steps of ethanol starting with 70%. From the blocs cylinder-biopsies were taken with a diamond cutting tool according to a drawing in which the topography of the cross-section was documented. The biopsy samples were ground with corrundium paper by hand using a wet grinding procedure.

The series of cross-sections could be digitalized via an interactive image analysis and three dimensionally reconstructed thereafter. Eight different compartments could be differentiated and reconstructed independently using a subtraction procedure. Thus, clear characterization of the type of anchorage of the implants could be worked out. Due to these three-dimensional displays the different anchorage principles could also be clearly distinguished.

2.3.2
Summary of Results

In cemented stems four anchorage types were defined. For that both the stiffened spongiosa and the completeness of the cement sheath were considered as essential.

If the spongiosa was preserved in the proximal femur and was stiffened in the U-shape of load transmission the bone showed no atrophy. If a connective tissue-free bone-to-cement interface was demonstrated, and the cement sheath was not destroyed, even after ten, eleven or twenty years, in this case a proximal anchorage was considered, even if fibrous tissue had developed in the stem's distal third (Figs. 22–25).

The proximal anchorage revealed in all cases failures of the medullary canal's drainage during insertion of bone cement and stem, thus the distal shape of the cement sheath is round indicating hydraulic pressure acting on it (Fig. 22). The sequence of sections displays proximally fibrous tissue free bone-to-cement contacts (Fig. 23). In the stem's distal half tangential orientation of the adjacent trabeculae are apparent; around the tip fibrous encapsulation is pronounced and the cement sheath is microfractured towards its anterior and lateral wall (Fig. 24).

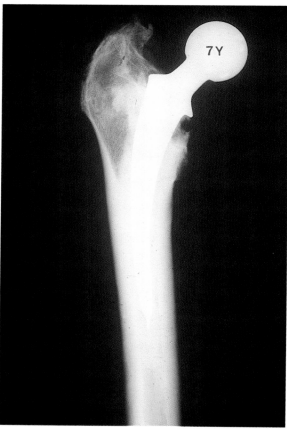

Fig. 22. Proximal anchorage of a Müller "banana" 7 years after implantation. Except an osteolysis along Adam's arch due to HDPE wear, no lucent line is visible. The round shape of the distal cement sheath and the gap between cement and bone indicate maldrainage of the canal; thus fluid and bone marrow has been forced hydraulically into the interface

2.3 Histomorphology of Human Samples

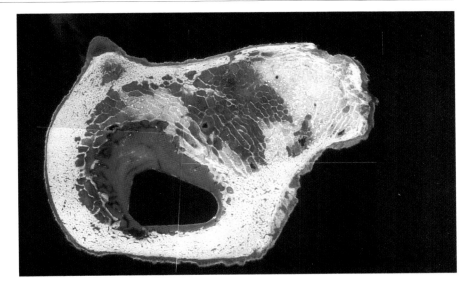

Fig. 23. Fibrous tissue-free contacts at the level of the minor trochanter and an intact cement sheath

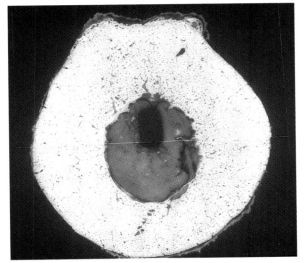

Fig. 24. Cross-section of the tip level with microfractures in the cement directed towards both the anterior and lateral walls

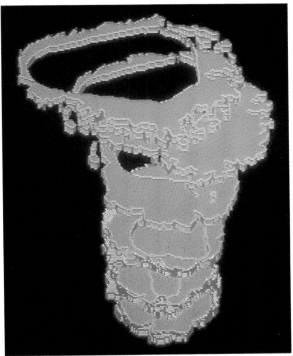

Fig. 25. Three dimensional reconstruction of the cement sheath with display of the proximal firm anchorage and the distal fibrous encapsulation. Blue line, fibrous tissue layer

The type of the anchorage is best shown in a three-dimensional reconstruction of the intact cement sheath together with the fibrous tissue. Quite obviously the loosening starts distally, thus representing a proximal anchorage type (Fig. 25). A bony anchorage of the entire cement sheath was pronounced if the cancellous bone had been preserved at least in some compartments along the tube of the diaphysis and if that spongiosa was stiffened with bone cement, a complete bony anchorage showed no lucent line, no fibrous tissue in the interface and nearly no remodeling of the cortex except a thickening of the lateral wall's distal third. The offset was measured below 40 mm and cementation revealed a whiteout around the stem's proximal two third. The smart "Banana" stem was firmly anchored even without complete cementation of the metal tip (Figs. 26–29).

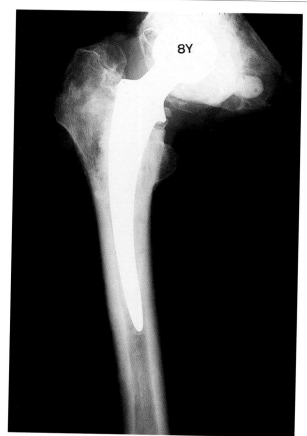

Fig. 26. Completely bony integrated Müller "banana" stem 8 years after implantation

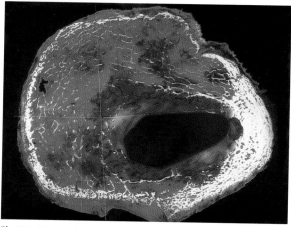

Fig. 27. Except for a circumscribed osteolysis with debris, a bony integration of the cement sheath is revealed

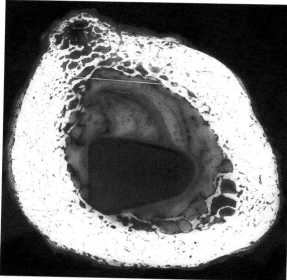

Fig. 28. Cross-section of the middle shaft level with bone contacts, partly stiffened cancellous bone and nearby remodeling in the cortex

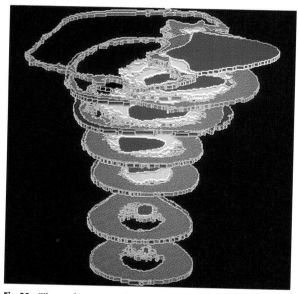

Fig. 29. Three-dimensional display without fibrous tissue over whole length of the stem. *Red*, stem; *yellow*, bone cement; *blue*, bone; *violet*, fibrous tissue)

If the stiffening was poor proximally, cement fragmentation and fibrous connective tissue could be seen; changes that decreased distally if a complete distal cement sheath existed, especially if peripherally preserved cancellous bone had been stiffened. In this case a distal bony anchorage could be described.

The distal anchorage shows a fibrous encapsulation proximally and a firm bone integration towards its distal implant bed (Figs. 30–33).

The self-locking cemented straight stem, the so-called cemented press-fit anchorage principle, lead in all

2.3 Histomorphology of Human Samples

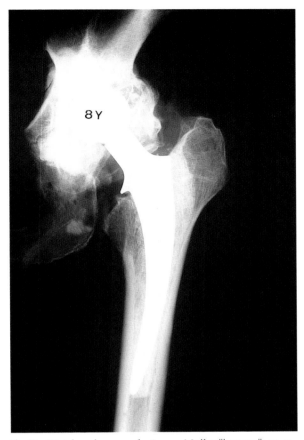

Fig. 30. Distal anchorage of a 8-year Müller "banana"; no radiolucent line is pronounced

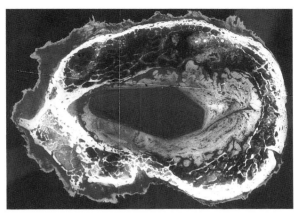

Fig. 31. A fibrous tissue sheath surrounds the cemented implant proximally; no bone contact is visible

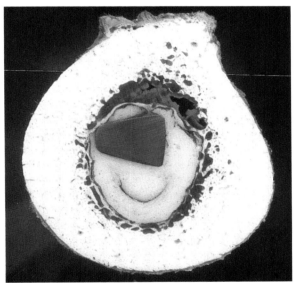

Fig. 32. The imcomplete cement sheath is bony integrated. Strong bone trabeculae support the implant. Bone is found directly on the metal surface

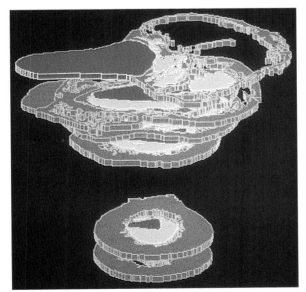

Fig. 33. Distal anchorage with thick fibrous tissue layers proximally and bony support distally. *Red*, stem; *yellow*, bone cement; *violet*, fibrous tissue; *blue*, bone

cases to the self-destruction of the cement sheath. The metal-to-bone load transfer destroyed the bone cement, the subsidence principle splits the cement sheath. The cement degradation was more pronounced proximally inducing a granuloma penetrating the interface. The three-dimensional reconstruction classified the type of anchorage as "cement press-fit" (Figs. 34–37). In nearly all samples the calcar femoris was completely or partly destroyed and in most cases the neck of the femur was resected.

Chapter 2 Histomorphology of the Bone-to-Cement Contact

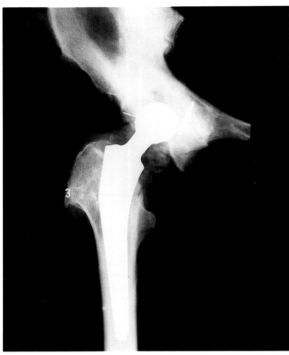

Fig. 34. Cemented press-fit stem (Müller straight or self-locking stem) 8 years after implantation. No radiolucent line is visible

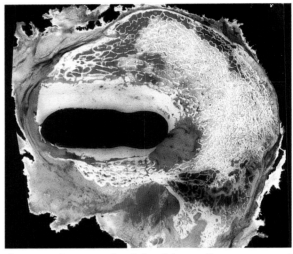

Fig. 35. A split cement sheath, breakdown of bone cement, and invasive granuloma emphasize the destruction process of this cementation principle

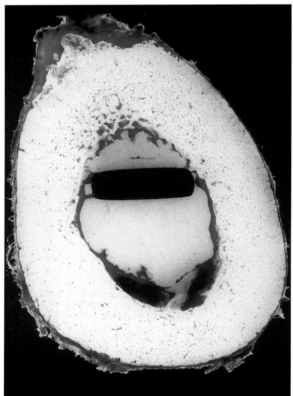

Fig. 36. Split cement sheath and thick granulomatous fibrous tissue around the implant

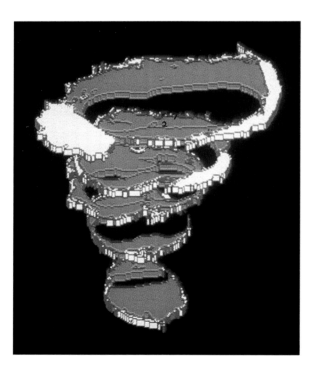

Fig. 37. Three-dimensional reconstruction of the destroyed cement sheath

CHAPTER 3
Can Cancellous Bone Carry the Load?

3.1
About the Deformation Behavior of Spongiosa

Compact bone reacts to an implant only if extended absorption along the Haversian systems reaches the interface. In order to analyze fine differences in the bony reaction of the bed with standardized implants, one must implant in an epiphysial cancellous bone bed.

Although the bone, with its macro-, micro and ultrastructure, has an anisotropic shape, the basic stress and strain relationship is valid.

3.1.1
Elasticity

Cancellous bone is structured in a way that resembles a shell more than a trabecula (Fig. 38). The living spongy bone is of elastic material which means that the framework of the bone deforms under load, and this deformation regresses after the load has been removed. The

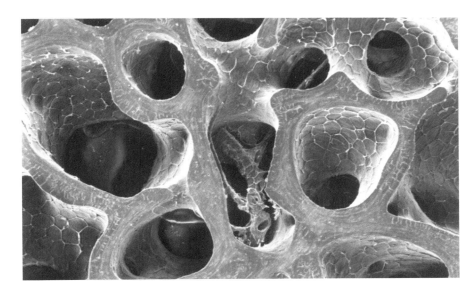

Fig. 38. Cancellous bone honeycomb in the tibial head of a dog. Spongious bone is structured in a way more resembling a shell than a trabecula. SEM of a frontal section

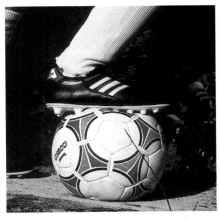
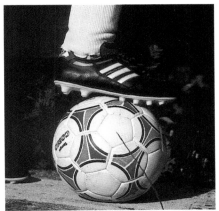

Fig. 39. The deformation of cancellous bone as demonstrated by Frost (1973)

Fig. 40. Restoration of the ball's shape after the load has been removed

ball underneath the foot (Figs. 39, 40) illustrates this clearly. The concept of elasticity does not indicate how fast the structure regains its original form. Around an implant cancellous bone is deflected at the interface (Fig. 41).

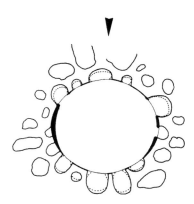

Fig. 41. Deflection of cancellous bone at the bone-to-implant interface under load: contact supports and gaps express a complicated deformation pattern

Hook's law determines the relation between stress and strain. As long as solid bodies react proportionally to each other, they belong to the category of Hookean materials. If the strain increases more than the stress, the materials do not follow Hook's law any longer. In a certain range of stress and strain, bone can be categorized as Hookean material. Thus $\varepsilon = k\sigma$ with ε representing the strain, k representing the proportionality factor and σ representing the stress form the equation $\varepsilon = k\sigma$. Bones represent complex biological structures. They do not only differ in their formation and composition of fibers, of ground substance and of mineral crystals, but they can also substantially differ in the arrangements of these components to each other. Because of the complex structure of bones, the physicist's exact way of looking at can only approximately grasp the complex process of the stress-strain relationship of bones.

The E modulus (Young's modulus) gives the relation of stress to strain, more precisely it gives the relation of the actual result of the stress divided by the actual result of the elastic deformation (strain): $E = \sigma/\varepsilon$. Thus the E modulus defines the stiffness of a material, which is the resistance against the deformation under an applied load. The higher the E modulus the stiffer the material.

The stiffness of an anisotropic material, as the spongiosa bone demonstrates, depends on the ultra- and microstructures, on the architecture of the framework of cancellous bone, on its mineralization and density and its arrangement of fibers. Finally it also depends on the composition of fibers, the intercellular substance and the hydration of the tissue. In the same way the stiffness depends, from a biological point of view, on the inner pressure, consisting of the proliferation pressure, the cells that fill in the spongiosa honeycomb, the turgor and the viscosity of cell contents (i.e., fat cells), of the intravascular pressure of the marrow sinusoid, of veins and arteries as well as of the osmotic and colloid osmotic pressures of the tissue. In conclusion, it depends also on the stress-strain relationship in fluids.

3.1.2
Viscoelasticity

The term viscoelasticity means that solid bodies (mostly polymers) deform gradually and increasingly under a constant load. In other words, relatively weak van der Waal's bonds break and chain-molecules slide past each other. Increasing temperature accelerates this effect. Viscoelastic behavior includes the regression of the deformation when the load is removed. This might take a long time and hardly reaches the initial dimensions. The materials miss resilience under static test conditions. Some polymers, however, show very good resilience under fast deformation conditions, for example rubber. Bone can demonstrate viscoelastic properties when loaded to its upper limit (Frost 1973).

3.1.3
Isotropic Deformation

Isotropic deformation does not characterize most materials, including bone. Only very few materials demonstrate it. Therefore the E modulus of bone changes not only with regard to load, but also due to its architecture, according to the direction in which it is tested, and also depending on its actual physiological state, for example the state of initial tension due to a hydraulic pressure.

Due to the architecture of the cancellous bone framework, and without taking into account the differences in material or in the initial tension of individual honeycombs, the anisotropic deformation can be demonstrated in a foam material with differently sized pores that is given a load. The deformation is the most significant where the largest pores and thus the least stiffness at equal wall-strength exist.

Regarding the deformation of anisotropic materials, bone has different elasticity moduli in different directions, i.e., different stiffness depending on direction.

3.1.4
Resilience and Damping

The deformation of a perfectly elastic material completely regresses ($\Delta L = 0$).

Among the dynamic parameters that characterize materials, resilience is the most important dimension. Resilience indicates how much energy of the mechanical

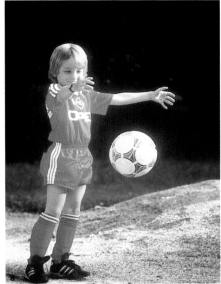 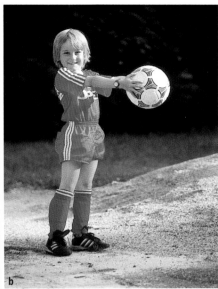

Fig. 42a,b. A soccer ball dropping to the ground becomes dented and springs back. It regains nearly the same height

work that is necessary to deform elastic material can be stored and restored. The resilience R equals the work W–ΔW (dissipated energy) divided by W. The smaller ΔW, the better the resilience of the material. When restoring its outer form, a perfectly resilient material transmits back all the mechanical energy that has been put into it in order to deform it. A soccer ball that drops to the ground from a certain height gets dented and springs back. It regains nearly the same height from which it fell due to the restoration of its original form (Fig. 42a, b).

3.1.5
Damping

The damping is also a dynamic parameter and represents the opposite of resilience. Damping indicates that a deformed material does not gain back its original form with the same amount of energy that the deformation used. This means the material transmits part of the mechanical work (energy) which was invested in it in order to deform it, into different forms of energy ("dissipation of strain energy").

Hydrated bone forms a better damping material under these circumstances than dry bone because a good part of the deformation energy is dissipated during the viscoelastic deformation, for example as heat or other forms of energy (hysteresis energy). The hydrated and the dehydrated dry bone react elastically in a broad mean of their stress-strain curve. Thus hydrated tendon and the very aqueous cartilage represent good damping materials. In a similar way to the resilience modulus, one can formulate a damping modulus where ΔW represents the work lost in different energies, work of the energy which was needed to deform and that did not transform back into the same mechanical energy of the system.

In comparison with the soccer ball as a nearly perfect resilient element that almost completely regained the height of drop, a lead ball represents a good damping material. By absorbing the deformation energy of free fall, the lead ball gets permanently deformed. The damping modulus: D = ΔW/W.

3.1.6
Breaking (Tensile) Strength and Toughness

Bone is a good example that toughness and tensile strength are completely different definitions. The strength represents the force in form of a load or a tension that causes a solid body to break. The toughness represents the complete deformation energy (mechanical work) that is necessary to break the body. Wet bone has a very high strength, in its vital state, but it has a much higher toughness. From a physics point of view, the force that causes a dry bone to break can be very high; however, the path that this breaking process covers is very short, so that the complete deformation energy is smaller than with a wet bone. The force to break a wet bone is possibly as high, but the path that the breaking process covers is much longer because the toughness, for example in the bending load, is much greater which results in the necessity of a much higher deformation energy in order to cause it to break.

3.1.7
Compliance

Compliance is a very important term if one wants to understand the dynamic processes of bones. Compliance represents the ability of a material or structure to give way or to deform especially under a dynamic load. The E modulus expresses the stiffness, and compliance represents the time dependent deformation. The higher the E modulus the lower the compliance. Few exact studies regarding the compliance of bone have been carried out to date. However, it is known that the compliance decreases substantially under sudden load and that a higher E modulus for the bone occurs. The equation of the quasi static compliance could be $C = 1/E$.

Under conditions of cyclic loading as it appears in the interface of endoprostheses the dynamic compliance equals the acceleration produced per unit of applied loading force and plays a more important role than E moduli under static conditions. Some properties in time-dependent terms of the dynamic compliances have not been considered adequately till now.

3.1.8
Energy

Energy represents an amount of mechanical work or any measurable equivalent amount of any other kind of energy expenditure; in terms of bone response it is important to know that mechanical energy can dissipate in other forms of energy thus inducing different tissue reaction. If for instance mechanical energy generated by muscle fibers acting on the bone-to-implant interface dissipates in kinetic energy, relative motion is generated inducing bone reabsorption and fibrous tissue formation.

3.1.9
Impact

Impact is an important dynamic quantitative unit of force which is of growing significance for the interpretation of the reaction of bone. Impulse represents the force acting on a body during a period of time. Thus, from an empirical point of view, one knows that the bone response fails to appear below a certain amount of one of the two factors: force or time. However, for example, with a certain amount of time bone remodeling activities take place under minor changes in force. The equation is defined as follows: $I = F\,t$

Rubin and Lanyon (1987) demonstrated that only the intermittent deformation, or the dynamic load, leads to "adaptive bone remodeling." Here, the impulse can be very short and its impact can be directly proportional to the degree of achieved deformation. In their experiments the authors came to the conclusion that the local differences in the response to the functional stimuli were genetically programmed. According to them, any deviation from the "optimal strain environment" would lead to an adaptive reaction of bone, either through growth or loss of mass.

Increasingly more importance is attributed to the essential variance of bone density and of the broad spectrum of anisotropy (Goldstein et al. 1983; Ciarelli et al. 1986; Goldstein and Matthews 1991). As a result of their computer-tomographic high-resolution-studies of cancellous bone sections, Goldstein et al. (1983) found a good correlation between the density and the mechanical characteristics of the spongiosa bone. In very systematic animal experiments they confirmed the adaptation of bone to controlled deformations.

3.2
Deformation of Bone Through Different Implants

If an implant is inserted in a spongy bed the continuous spongiosa architecture around the implant is interrupted, thus producing an interface, even if the implant is press-fit implanted and in contact with the bony bed. All trabeculae in contact with the implant experience primarily a deformation due to the press-fit implant. This static deformation deforms the spongiosa in accordance with its anisotropical structure.

During the transmission of force from the implant to the bone the surface structure of the implant turned out to be of essential importance. In addition to the static load, a dynamic load, applied directly or indirectly from the musculature, is acting on the bone structure deflecting it at the interface. The spongiosa honeycombs and trabeculae are deformed at the implant if its E modulus is higher than that of the corresponding bone compartment; otherwise the implant is deformed by the bone (i.e., silastic implants).

Due to these phenomena, highly complex deformation patterns occur around the implant. These are shown in a schematic and simplified way in Fig. 41. If the implant's Young's modulus is higher than that of the corresponding bone, a force which is transmitted through the bone to the implant is more or less completely reflected at an implant's rough surface. This mechanical energy is reflected in form of deformation work. At smooth surfaces, part of the mechanical energy dissipates due to shear stresses into kinetic energy producing relative motion; relative movements induce loss of mineral, bone reabsorption, and fibrous tissue formation. Repair mechanisms with new formation of immature woven bone result in a high turnover rate.

As a result of deflection at a 100 μm-rough surface the bone response reveals trabecular support without interposition of fibrous tissue, a reinforcement of all cancellous bone trabeculae throughout the epiphysis and a low turnover rate (Fig. 43).

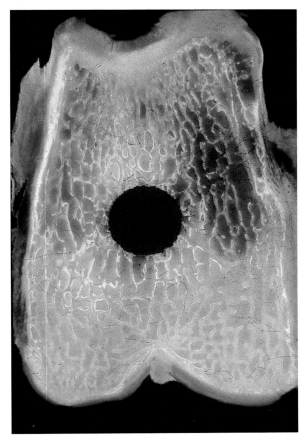 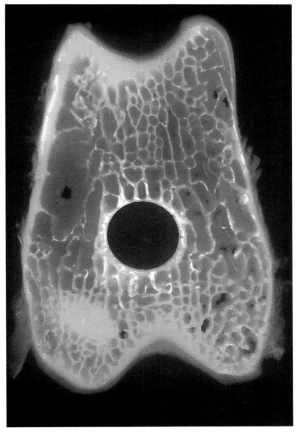

Fig. 43. Trabecular support of the rough titanium implant with reinforcement of the cancellous bone trabeculae throughout the epiphysis

Fig. 44. Fibrous and bony encapsulation of the titanium implant with a smooth surface

At a smooth surface part of the mechanical energy from load dissipates into kinetic energy thus inducing high bone turnover at the interface, fibrous and bony encapsulations of the implant due to relative motion (Fig. 44; Draenert and Draenert 1992; Breusch 1993).

Similar bone reactions are observed around femoral components i.e., the bony support of the tip of the femoral stem, seen in X-rays, which is in accordance with results of other experiments (Goldstein 1987; Goldstein and Matthews 1991). Frost (1987) describes the mechanism that regulates the bone mass as "mechanostat." He believes that signals of mechanical deformation control both the growth and the design of bone and remodeling because a specific relative deformation leads to bone renewal, and a decrease in impulses, with an absence of dynamic deformation, activates osteoclasts and leads to the decomposition of bone substance. Brighton et al. (1991) found increased concentrations of prostaglandin E2 in cell cultures during experiments on cell deformation. Other authors, including Hastings and Mahmud (1988) and Hasting et al. (1989), made good progress in measuring the so-called "strain-related potentials," or "strain-generated potentials," during the deformation of bone explained by a "streaming potential mechanism"; studies that differ somewhat from the classical piezo-electricity theory. However, no convincing studies in this active bone field have yet been carried out.

Studies by Scott and Korostoff (1990) classified these electrical potentials as signals for the remodeling process. A whole series of material testing of fresh, moist, and dry spongiosa bone was conducted. Some of these test results are certainly interesting with regard to the anisotropy of the spongy bone. For example, controlled studies by Linde et al. (1990) measured the breaking strength and the stiffness of the cancellous bone in three different axes and differentiated the elastically stored energy and the transmission into viscoelastic energy (hysteresic energy); this would not have been possible in standard breaking tests.

As with all mechanical measurements of dead, wet or dry bone samples, with or without bone marrow components, more or less disconnected from their environment, with open or cut off spongiosa honeycombs, tested on a smooth or rough test surface, these studies can only give information about the "bone" material and not about the organ "bone." There are many findings supporting the theory that the organ "bone" is hydraulically strengthened.

Since Evans and King (1961) had conducted such measurements of breaking strength with cubes of different spongiosa sections, details of the energy absorption of different spongiosa sections exist. However, this knowledge can be used only as a starting point for interpretation of in vivo situations. There is a discrepancy between the histological findings and calculated presumptions. However, a positive correlation could be established between the Young's modulus and the work carried out to break a structure; although the absolute data are certainly not precise, a trend can be demonstrated (Hvid and Jensen 1984; Hayes and Carter 1976; Hayes and Black 1979). Taking into consideration such significant differences in test designs and measurement arrangements of dead material it is not surprising that contradictions occur (McElhaney 1966). The basic biological mechanisms of the breaking strength of bone, especially under conditions of cyclic loading, play a significant role in resilience and compliance of bone. Therefore, studies evaluating the material under cyclic load as performed by Walker et al. (1976), Linde et al. (1985) and Radin et al. (1970) must be considered.

From histological results of a study with standardized implants with different roughness (Draenert and Draenert 1992; Breusch 1993), one can summarize that spongiosa gets "loading energy" transmitted through the musculature, via ligaments, tendons and capsule and by direct joint pressure. Furthermore, for the most part this energy gets stored as elastic energy by the spongiosa bone, and by restoring its form this energy is freed again as elastic energy with some lost energy (hysteresic energy). This energy, as the difference between "loading energy" and "unloading energy," dissipates in other forms of energy, for the most part in viscoelastic energy but certainly also in form of heat (Frost 1983; Linde and Hvid 1989).

In a pressfit inserted implant in the cancellous bone bed potential energy loaded i.e., by the musculature in the structure of the bone framework is transmitted to the implant or reflected off the implant. The energy is given back almost completely to the bone framework as elastic energy, precisely when Young's modulus of the implant is higher than that of the according bone bed. The energy transmission from bone to implant depends significantly on the surface roughness of the implant and the direction of the forces acting on it. In addition, we must take into consideration that a central defect itself absorbs part of the deformation energy by being deformed around the implant (Fig. 41). Since a large part of the deformation energy gets transmitted to the spongiosa framework by directed load through joint pressure, musculature, ligament and the capsule, this energy gets converted in some areas into kinetic energy around the implant, thus producing a gap. Tension stresses occur in the marrow honeycombs along the interface inducing meaningful signals for the pluripotential mesenchymal cells. These signals may trigger i.e., the production of collagen fibrils or stimulate even osteoclasts depending on the relative deformation of the cells (Perren and Cordey 1977). Layers of connective tissue of variable extent develop to stabilize the zone of relative motion. The extent depends on the deformation of the bone compartment.

Formation of fibrous tissue tangentially oriented to the implant's surface, quickly formed woven bone and ossification of collagenous fiber bundles limit relative movements to such an extent that "bone healing" can occur. These processes continue if an implant's smooth surface hinders stable anchoring of bony supports. Under that condition a high turnover rate of immature newly formed bone and finally fibrous and bony encapsulation appear. The high turnover rate and the frame formation (bony encapsulation) around the implant are expressions of this relative motion (Fig. 44).

Only with rough implant surfaces, where shear stresses do not lead to relative motion in the interface, is a large part of the deformation energy transmitted from the implant back to the bone framework: partly directly reflected and partly transmitted to other bone areas in form of elastic energy. According to Rubin and Lanyon (1987), cyclic impulses lead to the lamellar-concentric reinforcement of the cancellous bone trabeculae.

Direct adhesion onto the implant by covering the surface tangentially with mature lamellar bone can be demonstrated histologically with hydroxyapatite coated implants. It leads to direct transmission of laoding energy from bone to implant and vice versa. The bony structures are reinforced in the same way.

In addition to the classical studies concerning the relationship between the density of bone and the load acting on it (Pauwels 1965; Kummer 1963), new studies (Alho et al. 1988; Turner 1989) show as well that a clear correlation exists between the breaking strength of bone and its density. From standardized animal experiments over 1 year, one can conclude that in implants with a smooth surface a large part of the deformation energy is transmitted into relative motion in the interface; a high turnover rate yielded a bony encapsulation, and between implant and bone ring a fibrous tissue layer had formed. Three-dimensional analysis of the newly formed bone clearly shows that the density of bone directed toward the depth of the epiphysis increases. Density is highest where the bottom of the implant supports itself in the epiphyseal spongiosa. Bony supports are directed to the dorsal bone cortex (Fig. 45). From the direction of these trabecular structures a resultant is de-

3.2 Deformation of Bone Through Different Implants

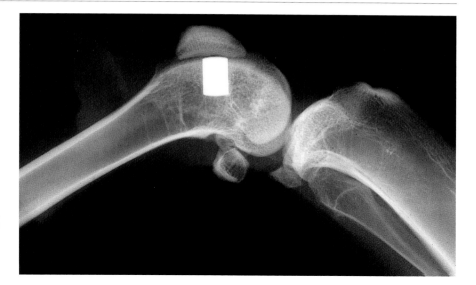

Fig. 45. Smooth titanium implant in the standardized defect of the patellar groove in the lateral view of an X-ray; bony support of the implant towards the dorsal femoral wall is revealed

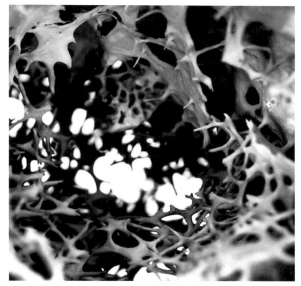

Fig. 46. Spongiosa resembles a shell much more than a trabecula; view upon the metaphyseal cancellous bone of the proximal femur

termined which is directed from proximal-ventral to caudal-dorsal and which corresponds very precisely to the diagonal longitudinal axis of the implant.

On the other hand implants with a rough surface or implants with a hydroxyapatite coated surface do not show this phenomenon to such an extent. These findings from the animal experiments correspond to the fibrous and bony encapsulation around prostheses components in human pathology (Draenert and Draenert 1992).

The conclusion that can be drawn is: Spongiosa resembles much more a shell (Weidenreich 1922) than a trabecula (Fig. 46)

In order to take into account the deformability of cancellous bone one can either develop isoelastic implants which might be difficult due to the anisotropy of the bone, or one can stiffen the spongiosa, e.g., by using bone cement. An empty egg breaks under a load of 2 kg, while an egg that has been stiffened with cooled bone cement via a needle tolerates this load without apparent deformation (Fig. 47).

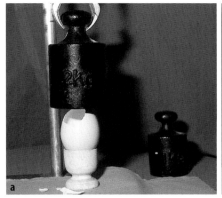 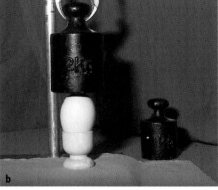

Fig. 47. a An empty egg breaks under the load of 2 kg. **b** An egg stiffened with bone cement resists to the same load without visible deformation

3.3
Stiffening of Spongiosa with Bone Cement

3.3.1
Human Histopathological Key Findings

In long lasting components of human beings it was always found that spongiosa bone had been preserved and had been stiffened with bone cement at least in some compartments. This experience was made with stem prostheses in the femur, components of knee prostheses, and Wagner resurfacing cups. In these cases histology confirmed connective tissue-free bone-to-bone cement contacts.

It was concluded: the success of cemented components was in all cases based on stiffened bone structures.

It is amazing that interest in the stiffness of the spongiosa bone came to the fore in connection with the artificial hinge-free knee joint replacement. The loosening rates of these knee joint components were considered to stay in direct correlation to the axial strength of the bone trabeculae (Hvid et al. 1983). Different study groups tried to determine the stiffness and strength of the bone. Goldstein et al. (1983) determined the stress and strain curves with 1 cm cubes under single-axial compression. They observed differences in the strength of the cubes up to many times over ten. Hvid et al. (1983) tried to obtain results in static studies via determination of the "ultimate stress" out of the stress-strain relationship curve (Young's modulus). In addition, they tried to determine the absorption of energy in vitro via a material-testing machine. Finally they tried to compare them to in vivo measurements with the "osteopenetrometer" which they had developed. They too found significant differences between different measured locations within the tibial plateau. The spongiosa areas of the medial condyle showed the highest material firmness, and the measurements with the "osteopenetrometer" came close to the measurements with the Instron-instrument in the laboratory.

Repeatedly, researchers tried to determine the stiffness of bone through density measurements. During such studies the mineral density of the spongiosa bone was compared with the bending strength of the femur in axial breaking tests (Alho et al. 1988). Alho et al. found high correlations between the spongiosa density and the breaking strength of the femur. They found even better correlations by calculating the bone mass from cross-sections as it had been by Pauwels (1965). Relations between different degrees of bone mineralization and strength of the material were also demonstrated by Currey (1984). This author confirmed that a high mineralization degree correlated with a high E modulus; lower mineralization conditions correlated with increased toughness of the bone, a lower E modulus, and medium values of breaking strength. It is easy to see that bone with very high mineral density can nevertheless have a low breaking strength, for it is known that necrotic bone absorbs minerals quickly and demonstrates a very high mineral density but has a very low breaking strength. As long as no additional physiological parameters are included in determining the strength of bone, material tests of physical nature can only show tendencies but they cannot reflect the biological in vivo condition of bone.

Bone density and bone mass determinations can give some indications of the bone's stiffness depending on the resolution capability of the applied process (Rüegsegger et al. 1982). However, these measurements show only tendencies because essential physiological guiding-mechanisms which are most likely of hydraulic nature (Kafka 1983; Draenert and Draenert 1984) cannot be grasped.

Deformation of spongiosa bone probably has two aspects: according to Frost (1983) the postulation of "minimum effective strain" (MES) represents the attempt to define a deformation during which an apposition of bone occurs: according to Lanyon (1973) a continuous cyclic load to the bone structure is necessary in order to maintain the existing mass. According to the author, decreasing load results in absorption and disuse atrophy of the bone and excessive load leads to the bone's reinforcement by apposition. It remains doubtful whether the definition of a "unit strain" (Frost 1983) without time dependence can define the stimulus of bone formation. The ideas of Lanyon (1973) concerning cyclic loading must be defined more precisely with regard to amplitude and time dependency, therefore further tests are needed which take into consideration impulses and specific energies. In this context, another aspect to be considered concerns the deformation of the spongiosa framework which can lead to connective tissue replacement or even to fatigue fracture of bone. The phenomenon is known from the anchorage of cement-free joint components (Haddad et al. 1986; Cook et al. 1991; Draenert 1988; Sychterz and Engh 1996) and can be understood as cyclic overloading.

In all femoral components stably anchored for years cancellous bone was preserved and stiffened by an inlet of bone cement (Figs. 22–33). Higher magnifications revealed clearly the type of anchorage: "elephant feet" contacts stably supported the cement implant surrounded by bone marrow spaces (Fig. 48a); if, however, a row of honeycombs was not reinforced by bone cement a gap filled in with fibrous tissue was apparent. (Fig. 48b).

Clinical experience resulted in cementing PCA and Miller-Galante tibial components (Figs. 49, 50). It is not a coincidence that the results with respect to shifting and loosening of these components were much better than when implanting without bone cement. From a pure

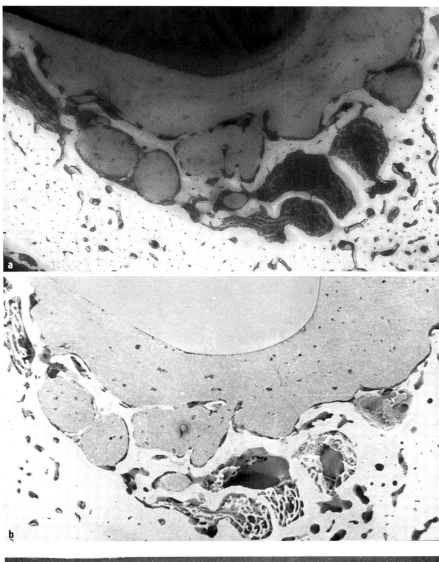

Fig. 48. a Interlocking of bone cement in the strong cancellous bone honeycombs along the tube of the femur. **b** Same specimen in the SEM demonstrating elephant feet contacts on the bone-to-cement interface while on the right side where no interlocking is seen a gap has formed between bone cement and bone

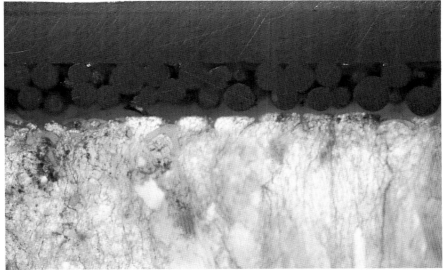

Fig. 49. A cement-free PCA tibial component. Window in the middle of the tibial plateau revealing stress shielding in the adjacent bone and fibrous tissue around the metal component. Two years and 3 months after implantation

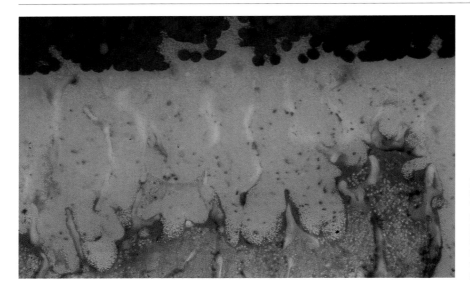

Fig. 50. A cemented Miller-Galante tibial component. Window in the middle of the tibial plateau revealing intact bony trabeculae embedded in bone cement; no fibrous tissue has formed. Nine weeks after implantation (Specimen: Fuchs, Bayreuth)

science perspective the individual spongiosa honeycomb was stiffened and could resist deformation through the bone cement filling. This had two enormous consequences on the bone framework: first, transmission of force resulted over broad areas of spongy bone, second, deformation was resisted which would have otherwise resulted in fatigue, absorption and connective tissue formation, or even in fatigue fracture of trabeculae. Human pathological studies and systematic animal studies were conducted concerning this phenomenon.

Findings on femoral heads which were equipped with Wagner cups, and results from animal experiments with apes during which Wagner cups were implanted accomplish the above documented histological findings. Open questions were evaluated with animal studies in rabbits, e.g., addressing the question whether spongiosa bone is damaged through bone cement filling, or whether spongiosa bone embedded in bone cement can survive.

3.3.2
Histomorphological Findings in the Proximal Femur After Joint Surface Replacement

In 1974 Wagner was the first to implant a cup prosthesis which he had developed himself (Wagner 1978). First the procedure was enthusiastically accepted in clinics, later it was abandoned. It was based on the surface replacement of the femoral head in connection with a thin walled HDPE cup while the two components were cemented. Parallel to Wagner, in 1974 Gerard implanted his first cement free "double cup" (Gerard 1978). A little later more modifications were added which, however, did not change the principle (Freeman et al. 1978; Tanaka 1978; Salzer et al. 1978; Tillmann and Thabe 1983).

After good results initially, the procedure was quickly discontinued due to high loosening rates and fractures. A stress analysis by Schreiber and Jacob (1984) found a stress concentration at the rim of the metal cup. The study by Huiskes et al. (1985) came to similar conclusions: stress concentration at the level of the cup's rim and a "stress shielding" in the remaining areas of the femoral head, more pronounced above the center of rotation.

The clinical results were generally bad (Head 1981; Jolley et al. 1982; Bell et al. 1985; Ritter and Gioe 1986). The histological studies, without exception, demonstrated connective tissue and bone atrophy under the cups (Schreiber and Jacob 1984; Delling et al. 1984; Claes et al. 1990).

Although many loosened hip heads seemed to confirm this result, it remained unexplained why others were worn without complaints for 12 years or more. This triggered a histological study of femoral heads which were equipped with a surface replacement and whose components were still solid (Bucholz 1992).

During these studies it became apparent that the spongiosa had not become atrophic where it was stiffened with bone cement. It had resisted deformation and was preserved over the years (up to 12 years) in solid contact to the implant without interposition of connective tissue.

The areas could be demonstrated in a preparation which had been implanted for 2 years (Fig. 51). The cancellous bone of the femoral head, medially and laterally, as revealed in the frontal section, has been stiffened by bone cement. The white fluorescence of bone trabeculae was nicely contrasted to the blue-green fluorescence of the synthetic material, and on the distal side of each trabecula bone marrow spaces were apparent. The spon-

3.3 Stiffening of Spongiosa with Bone Cement

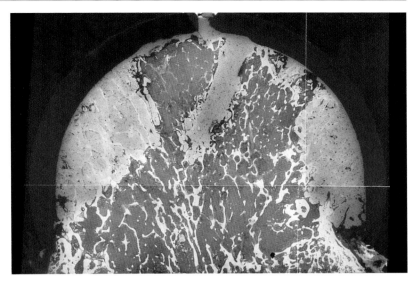

Fig. 51. Wagner cup 2 years after surgery: the stiffened spongiosa has not only remained alive but also has not atrophied; it shows impressively that it can resist deformation. Areas below the metal that were not stiffened have atrophied

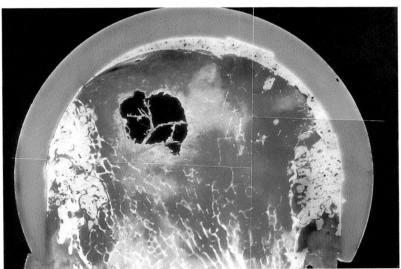

Fig. 52. Wagner cup 10 years after surgery: the areas where force was transmitted are stiffened and resistant. The unstiffened area has completely atrophied (stress shielding)

giosa was fully intact and vital. Immediately adjacent to the lateral stiffened area (on the left half of Fig. 51) an area that had not been stiffened with cement is revealed. The spongiosa structures still could be recognized morphologically as demineralized connective tissue beams, but they were completely atrophied. Adjacent to that area a cement plug had penetrated a drill hole forming a nonreinforced cement plug. There was a fibrous encapsulation of the cement implant visible, except in a small stiffened spongiosa area at the tip of the cement cone. Only this area showed connective tissue-free contacts. Medially another area was connected which once again was stiffened by bone cement and in which the beams were completely preserved in the way described above. The Wagner cup was absolutely solid and the scaffolding of cancellous bone was nearly unchanged. The same phenomena were confirmed in another, less completely cemented, case. Everywhere where the spongiosa honeycombs had been stiffened they resisted deformation. Where there were nonreinforced cementations connective tissue had formed, and where no stiffening existed atrophy and degeneration of bone occurred.

A Wagner cup 10 years after surgery gave another example. It showed stiffened spongiosa structures only around the cup's rim (Fig. 52). In this case the anchorage remained solid over the years, and only spongiosa structures of the femoral head which had been stiffened with bone cement have been preserved. The rest of the epiphyseal spongiosa has completely atrophied and could only be recognized by remaining connective tissue septation. Along the cement interface a very thin bone lamella had developed on the bone. The vessels' maintenance system, with strong muscular arteries, was completely intact and was demonstrated using a micromanipulator.

3.3.3
Histomorphological Findings on Cancellous Bone Stiffened with Bone Cement in the Distal Epiphysis of the Femur in Rabbits

The question of whether spongiosa enclosed in bone cement gets damaged by the bone cement and gets necrotic, or whether spongiosa atrophies and degenerates in the cement implant could only be answered with systematic animal experiments. Therefore, in animal experiments with rabbits bone cement was used to fill out the spaces of the spongiosa framework of the epiphyses of the patellar groove. This was done starting from a cylinder defect at the center of the patellar groove made by diamond cutters. Then, vacuum cannulae were inserted in both sides of the distal epiphysis. The defect in the patellar groove was closed with bone cement to the bony base plate of the cartilage, and the defect of the gliding surface to the cartilage was filled and modeled with bone wax. The animals were sacrificed after 35, 56, 84 days, and after 1 year, using a perfusion technique. After perfusion fixation through the abdominal aorta with Karnovsky solution a low viscosity resin was injected for casting the vasculature. During the first 5 weeks a continuous polychromatic labeling (Rahn and Perren 1971) was performed, beginning with the fifth postoperative day using the sequence oxytetracycline (yellow), alizarin complexon (red), calcein blue, calcein green, and oxytetracyclin.

Although the filling of epiphyseal spongiosa with bone cement is not always easy in animal experiments, successful embedding of wide areas of the spongiosa was achieved due to the vaccum technique (Fig. 53).

Cancellous bone trabeculae adjacent to bone cement did not show empty osteocyte lacunae weeks after surgery. Only a few spongiosa trabeculae, which have been fractured and which were torn out due to surgery followed by complete embedding in cement, showed partly bone necrosis. Bone adjacent to the bone cement implant was alive up to the interface. In thin sections osteocytes were observed up to the synthetic material. The spongiosa honeycombs were, for the most part, filled in completely with bone cement and were free of connective tissue. Polychromatic sequential labeling revealed that new bone had been formed in the gaps between the implant and the bone wall in the first weeks after surgery (Fig. 54). The gaps were completely filled in after the first 5 weeks. Bone had formed on both the implant and the spongiosa walls.

Higher magnification showed that newly formed bone had connective tissue-free contact with the implant. Living osteocytes were observed in contact with individual polymeric spheres of bone cement (Fig. 55).

Bone cement implants of the spongiosa honeycomb generally did not exceed a diameter of 1000 μm. They were, based on theoretical considerations, too small a mass of self-polymerizing substance to generate heat that would have lead to heat necrosis. With this in mind, it was amazing that live osteocytes could even be found in fragments embedded in bone cement. The fact that bone cement stiffened spongiosa honeycombs revascularize very quickly was shown early in experiments with apes in which castings of the vasculature were performed. The same experiments showed a highly complex bone cement shrinkage pattern with gaps and contact areas that formed in the cancellous bone framework embedded in the bone cement (Fig. 56). Polychromatic sequential labeling demonstrated that new bone formed here without delay, after a very quick revascularization, through the gaps between the implant and the bone. This

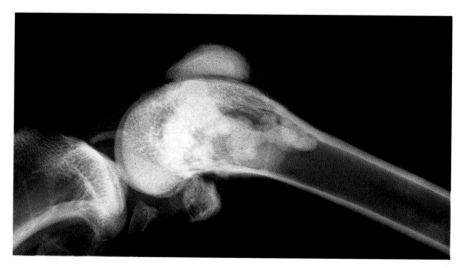

Fig. 53. Stiffening of the epiphyseal spongiosa of a rabbit using the vacuum technique; lateral view in the X-ray

3.3 Stiffening of Spongiosa with Bone Cement

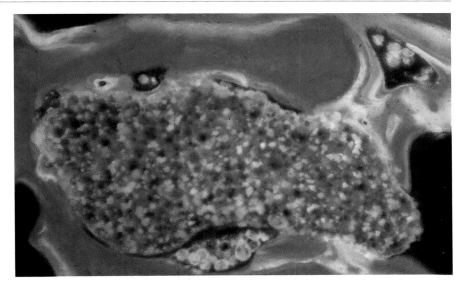

Fig. 54. Healing of the gap between bone and bone cement 5 weeks after the operation. Colors correspond to the bone forming activities: yellow, first week; blue, second week; red, third week; green, fourth week

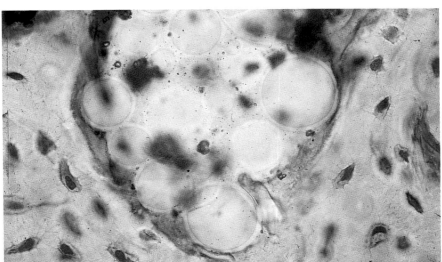

Fig. 55. Connective tissue-free contacts between single polymer beads and living osteocytes are revealed

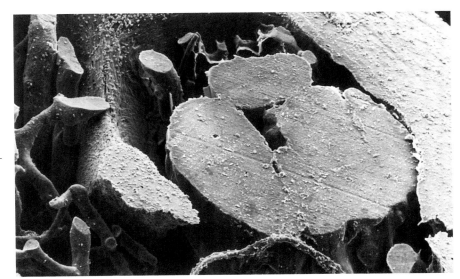

Fig. 56. Cancellous bone honeycombs filled with bone cement which has shrunken onto the bone on one side and away from the rest of the comb's wall thus creating a gap through which revascularization could take place. SEM of an ape's femoral head 9 months after the operation

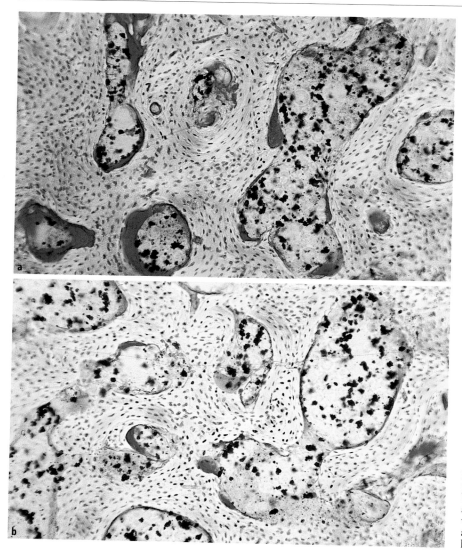

Fig. 57a,b. One year after implantation, an active symbiosis between bone cement and bone can be seen revealing secondary cavities and intact trabeculae with living osteocytes

newly formed bone is deposited both on the cement implant and on the walls of the bony bed. Load is distributed from the joint to the bone framework, transmitting loading energy through the bone trabeculae. Thus, bone is preserved, remodeling activities remain activated and disuse atrophy does not appear even after 1 year (Fig. 57).

The present results conclude that the spongiosa honeycomb architecture can be filled completely with bone cement without endangering the nourishment of the bone and without stress shielding effects. This might be different with cement implants in metaphyseal compartments because the load is introduced primarily to the epiphyseal cancellous bone, from which it can be transmitted to the cortex via a shunt of reinforced trabeculae. If so, the spongiosa embedded in bone cement in the metaphyseal compartment is no longer loaded, thus bone atrophies and is replaced by fibrous tissue (Bloebaum et al. 1984; Goodman et al. 1985)

The conclusions that can be drawn from basic and applied research are:

- Stiffened spongiosa can carry the load; it does not atrophy, and remains alive and reactive if embedded in bone cement.
- Cancellous bone must be preserved, washed out and filled with bone cement in areas where it is loaded.
- Preserved cancellous bone, washed out and filled in with bone cement does not show signs of heat.
- Only delicate and smart implants have been found among the positive long-term histological results; massive stems must be avoided.

- The retrotorsional momentum in the heel-strike phase must be opposed by a stabilizing structure: the femoral neck.
- The femoral neck must be preserved and the essential structure of the calcar femoris should not be damaged.
- Only an intact spongiosa can resist deformation. Only the open medullary cavity honeycomb can be filled with cement, and this only if blood coagulate and fat have been washed out using H_2O_2 (5%) and jet lavage.
- The bone rasp must be eliminated from the operating theater
- The instrument of choice is the diamond cutting tool as a wet grinding procedure.
- These results lead to a completely new operation technique which is close to that of Charnley's (1979) but due to validation of all different steps more reliable and more reproducible. Therefore we will go through the next chapters one step back to the future.

CHAPTER 4

Approach to the Hip Joint

For total hip replacements two different approaches have been widely introduced: (a) the posterolateral approach and (b) the transgluteal approach according to Bauer (1986).

4.1 Posterolateral Approach

Position the patient on his side firmly fixed from both sides anteriorly and posteriorly by adequate supports. The entire leg must be prepared and must be freely movable.

The incision starts two widths of a finger below and four proximal of the greater trochanter (GT) and is continued distally in an archlike fashion slightly anteriorly of the GT along the lateral side of the femur one width of four fingers (Fig. 58).

The subcutis is cut to the fascia lata. The fascia lata is split till the fibers of the musculus gluteus maximus are exposed; then they are separated atraumatically.

The leg is held in internal rotation during exposure of the small external rotator muscles.

The sciatic nerve is isolated and labeled by a silicon tube. The small rotators (musculus obturator internus et gemelli sup. and inf.) are tenotomized at the bone, labeled by a suture and retracted atraumatically, thus exposing the posterior capsule of the joint (Fig. 59).

The capsule is incised along the fossa interotrochanterica leaving the vascular area of the a. circumflexa medialis along the fossa intertrochanterica intact (Fig. 60). With a "T" incision through the labrum acetabulare the femur is exarticulated.

Fig. 59. Exposure of the sciatic nerve and incision of the small rotators

Fig. 60. "T" incision of the capsule leaving intact the arterial arch

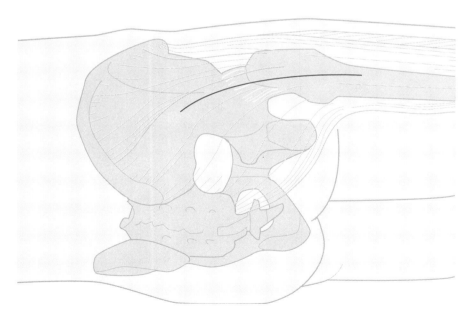

Fig. 58. Posterolateral approach. The incision starts two widths of a finger below and four proximal to the greater trochanter and is continued distally in an archlike fashion slightly anterior to the greater trochanter along the lateral side of the femur

4.1 Posterolateral Approach

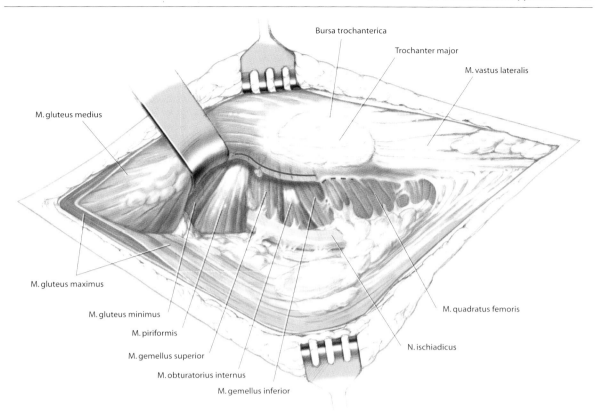

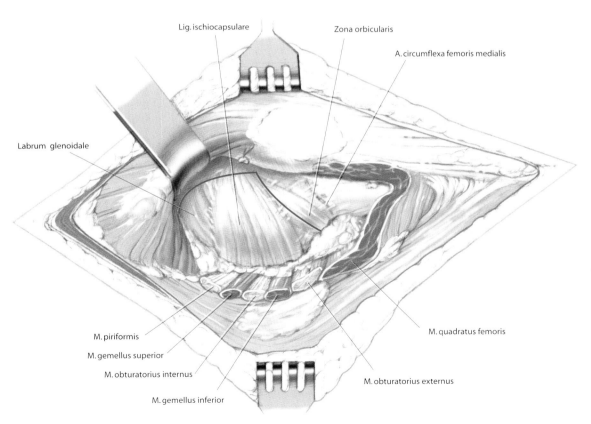

4.2
Transgluteal Approach

For the transgluteal approach (anterolateral approach, after Bauer 1986) the patient is positioned on his back, the clunis elevated and overlapping the operating table (Fig. 61). The incision is slightly concave towards the ventral side, one finger's width below the GT and from the tip of it four fingers' widths distally and proximally.

After incision of the subcutis and the fascia lata between the gluteus maximus muscle and the tensor fasciae latae parallel to the skin incision the gluteus medius muscle and the lateral vastus of the quadriceps are exposed. Sharp incision between the anterior and middle third of the muscle's portion to the bone and subperiosteal preparation of the musculature together with the tendoperiosteum keeping the osteotome close to the bone detach the musculature in one layer revealing the anterior capsule below (Fig. 62).

"T" cut of the capsule reveals a longitudinal incision oriented along the fiber bundles of the iliofemoral ligament and circularly connected incision parallel to the linea intertrochanterica, preserving the arterial blood supply from the ascendant branch of the arteria circumflexa lateralis (Fig. 63).

After cut of the labrum acetabulare the femoral head can be exarticulated supporting the greater trochanter with a Hohmann hook.

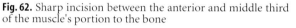

Fig. 62. Sharp incision between the anterior and middle third of the muscle's portion to the bone

Fig. 63. "T" cut of the capsule following the path of the fiber bundles of the iliofemoral ligament

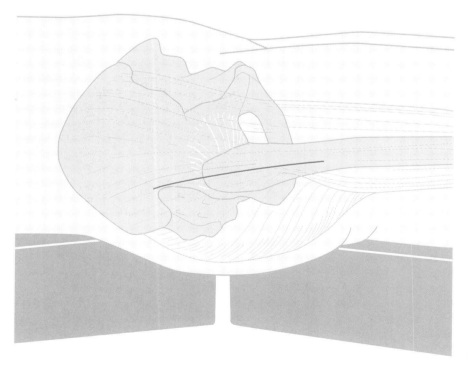

Fig. 61. Transgluteal approach according to Bauer (1986). Position of the patient, the clunis elevated, and overlapping the operating table

4.2 Transgluteal Approach

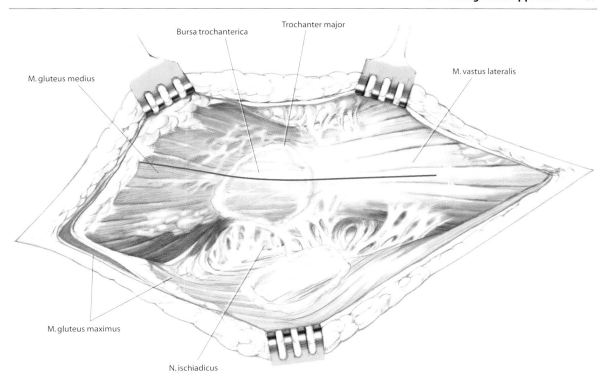

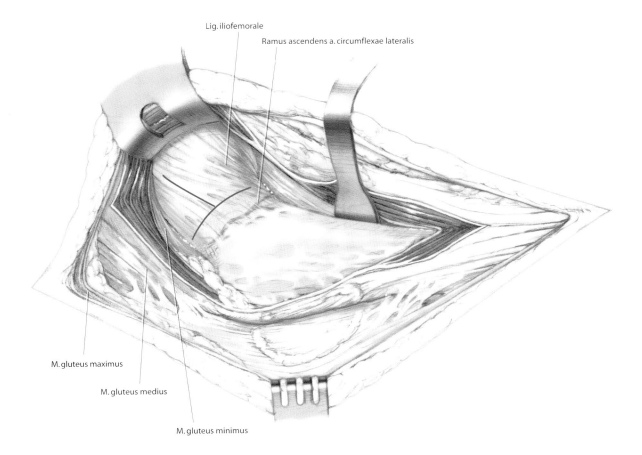

CHAPTER 5

Preparation of the Acetabulum

In many hospitals the femoral component of a hip arthroplasty is cemented but the acetabular component is used cement free [hybrid total hip reconstruction (THR)], mostly according to the press-fit principle; it is, however, pathohistologically verified, from surface replacement of the femoral head and the knee joint, that forces are transmitted through the rim of the cup, and that behind the cup a severe bony atrophy develops as time goes on (Draenert and Draenert 1992). Not all knowledge from studies on femoral components has been applied to the cementation technique of the acetabulum. Cementing the acetabulum must take into consideration that cement never should remain unconstrained, and should if ever possible be reinforced by bony structures, therefore the compact bone of the roof must be opened till the cancellous structure is freed.

In many cases a cement glance is produced by pressing an unflanged cup too hardly into the acetabulum without any distance holder.

Pathohistological studies of cup specimens resulted in three important findings: (a) The penetration of bone cement into the spongiosa of the pelvis was insignificant, (b) unlike in the femur, the cement was frequently cemented to a compact bone layer which was only pierced with anchorage holes that frequently showed sharp edges, (c) none of the studied samples showed any bony contacts around the anchorage plugs of the cement in the os pubis or os ischii. All anchorage cones were surrounded by broad resorption zones and thick connective tissue (Draenert 1986).

The result of the high-pressure technique (Lee and Ling 1981) in a perfect filling of the pelvis' cancellous bone honeycombs; it needs, however, special experience not to fill up too much of the structures of the iliac bone.

Laboratory tests on cadaver bones demonstrated that a vacuum set in the roof does not produce a negative-pressure in the os pubis or os ischii, and furthermore, even in the iliac bone no negative-pressure developed if the compact bone in the acetabulum was not partly removed. Opening it resulted immediately in a negative-pressure increase in the acetabulum (Draenert 1988). An even distribution of bone cement could only be achieved by thinning the compact bone with the spherical diamond grinder. Anchorage and deep drill holes led to

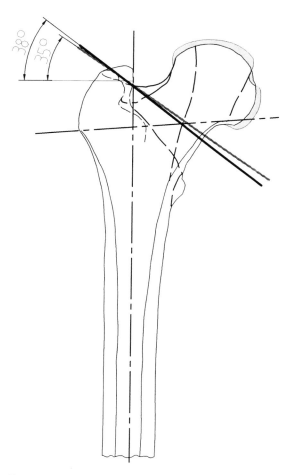

Fig. 64. Preservation of the neck prescribes an osteotomy of 35°–38°. The osteotomy starts from the transition of the neck to the greater trochanter

shunt connections of the vacuum: the cement was suctioned in directly through the anchorage tunnel into the suction cannula.

Positioning of two cannulae 1 cm above the superior lip of the acetabulum result in a perfect filling of the roof with bone cement up to the level of the cannula. This fact makes the filling of the pelvis' structures predictable.

5.1 Preparatory Steps

Before the acetabulum can be prepared the femoral head and neck has to be osteotomized preserving the neck: an inclination of 35°–38° meets that goals (Fig. 64).

5.2 Exposure of the Acetabulum

The first position is to prepare the inferior lip of the facies lunata using an ischial bone hook (Fig. 65). The inferior lip presents a sharp edge below which the ischium can be embraced by the ischial bone hook.

The second position is the exposition of the superior lip of the acetabulum. After exposure using a Hohman hook a drill guide is used (Fig. 66) to drill two 4.5-mm

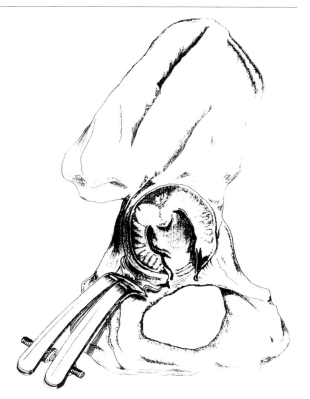

Fig. 65. The first position is to prepare the inferior lip of the facies lunata using the ischial bone hook

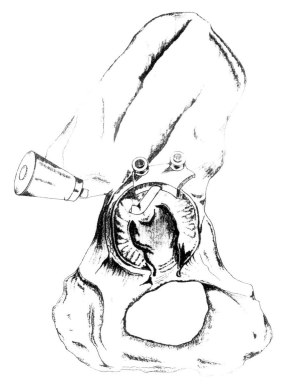

Fig. 66. After exposure of the superior lip of the acetabulum a drill guide for the two vacuum cannulae is used

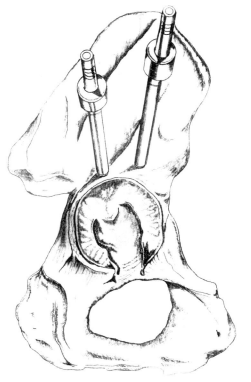

Fig. 67. Placement of two cannulae in the roof of the acetabulum

holes 1 cm above the roof with a distance of 2 cm into the iliac bone. Two cannulae are screwed in (Fig. 67), and obstructing debris is removed using a 2-mm K-wire. The two cannulae act as drainage cannula and as retractor as well.

5.3
Fossa Acetabuli

The cartilage is removed using a sharp spoon (Fig. 68). The fossa acetabuli should not be completely cleared from soft tissue because of bleeding which can occur.

5.4
Preparation of the Bony Acetabulum

The central part of the compact bone of the facies lunata, leaving intact its strong cortical rim, are thinned to its spongiosa structure using a wet grinding process with spherical diamond cutters (Fig. 69). The speed of the drilling machine should range from 1500–2000 rpm and the power should reach at least 300–400 W.

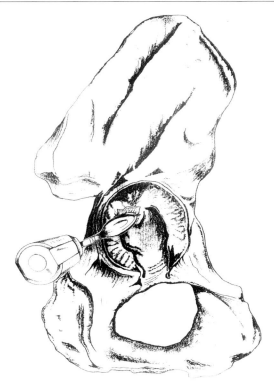

Fig. 68. The cartilage is removed using a sharp spoon

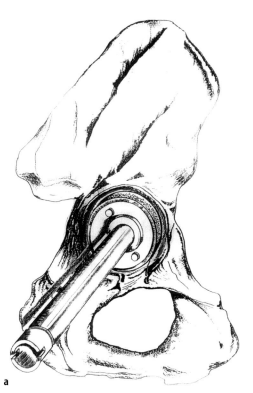

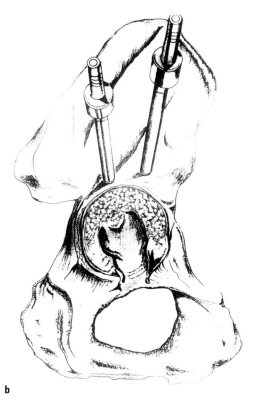

a
b

Fig. 69a,b. The central part of the compact bone of the facies lunata, leaving intact its strong cortical rim, is thinned using a diamond cutter

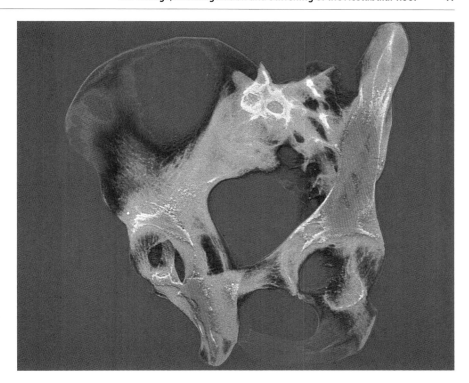

Fig. 70. The supporting roof of the acetabulum clearly shows the dense spongiosa structures directed towards the sacroiliac joint

5.5
Anatomical Composition of the Joint Surface of the Acetabulum

The acetabulum clearly shows a composition of three joint surfaces (Tillmann 1981). Intersections between the os pubis and the ischial bone are still apparent in the normal basin. Pressure measurements during application of vacuum show that the inner compartments are separated: vacuum applied in the iliac bone has no effect in the os pubis or ischii (Draenert 1981). Considering relative movements between all three compartments under load, cementation of the pubical or ischial compartment of bone appears unwise.

The orientation of the cancellous bone structure is directed from the roof with inclination towards the sacro-iliac joint forming a weight bearing column (Fig. 70). The alignment of the center of rotation to the center of the sacroiliac joint is indicated by the bone structure itself.

5.6
Lavage, Anticoagulation and Stiffening of the Acetabular Roof

Bone cement can only be suctioned into the cancellous structures of the iliac bone when the honeycombs are carefully cleaned and freed from most of the fat, blood and debris.

First the compact bone is thinned using the diamond until the spongiosa structure is visible.

After having freed the central cancellous bone structure, the trial cup is inserted measuring 2 mm less than the last used diamond cutters. The jet lavage is then used, removing carefully all debris material. Ringer's solution is injected through the two cannulae and then 2.20 ml of a solution of 10,000 IU heparin in 300 ml Ringer. After working the bone of the acetabulum two compresses soaked in 5% H_2O_2 are placed in the cavity, and the two cannulae are linked to the vacuum pump. At half vacuum the acetabulum is dried. Bone cement is now ordered.

The cement which is mixed under vacuum is prepressurized and then suctioned into the spongiosa using a silicon seal after having removed the pads and increasing the vacuum to full power (Fig. 71). The bone cement reaches the level of the cannulae and does not penetrate further into the structure of the iliac bone (Fig. 72).

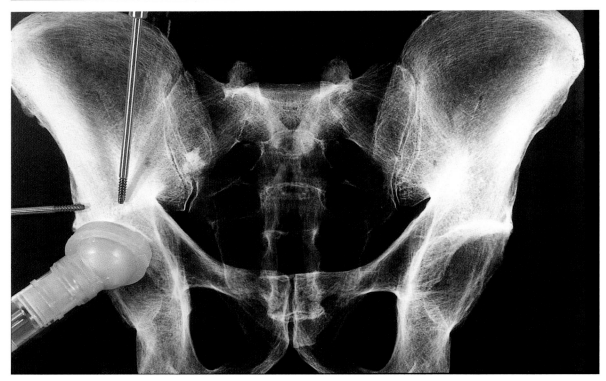

Fig. 71. The bone cement is suctioned into the iliac bone using a silicon seal hold against the acetabular roof

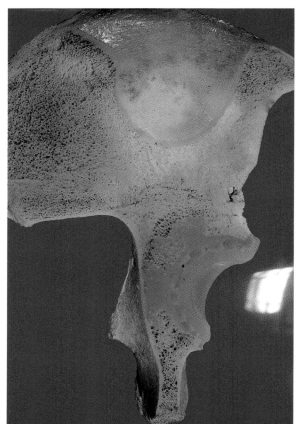

Fig. 72. Using vacuum application the bone cement can be suctioned free of artefacts to a predictable depth

5.7
Inclination and Alignment

Studies with cadaver specimens showed that large mediocaudal cement masses occurred between the cup and the acetabulum during the implantation of the cup if the lateral edge was inserted first and then the cup placed. Clinically investigated, big cement masses mediocaudally, were top heavy from the beginning and became loose at an early stage (Figs. 73, 74; Draenert 1983).

The cup should be inserted with the mediocaudal edge first, and placed with an inclination of 35°–40° and an anteversion of 12°. The mass distribution should be symmetrically aligned to the weight bearing structure directed to the sacroiliac joint (Fig. 75).

Using low vacuum during curing of the cement the cup does not have to be held in place because the blood is suctioned away and the cup remains firmly in place.

5.7 Inclination and Alignment

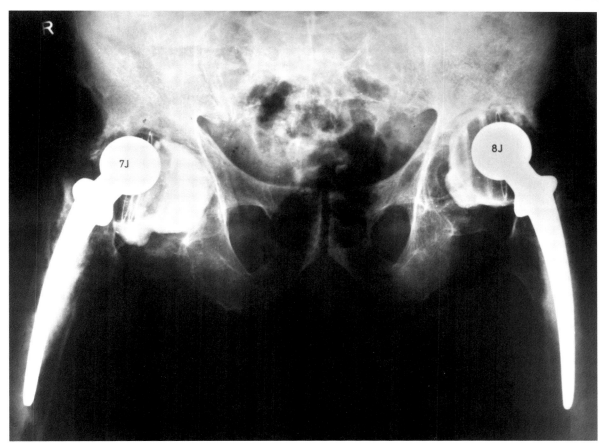

Fig. 73. Large cement masses medially and caudally are top-heavy from the beginning

Fig. 74a,b. Illustration of an equilibrium which becomes top heavy by an additional mass

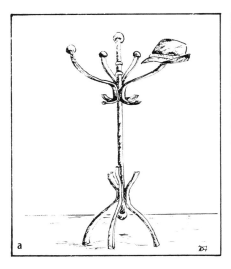 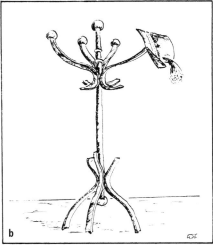

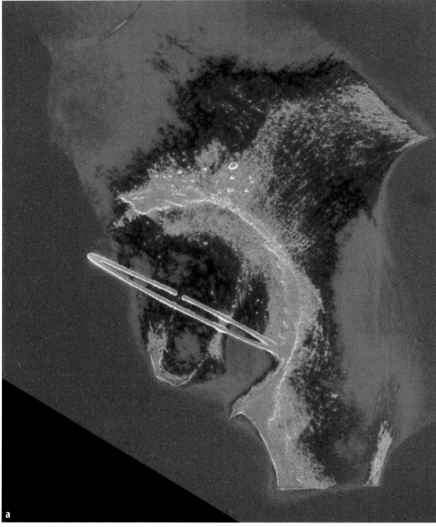

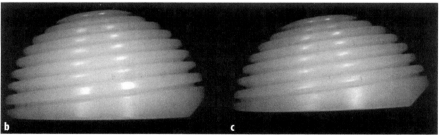

Fig. 75a. A 35° inclination of the cup, perpendicular to the resultant force which is directed to the sacroiliacal joint. **b,c.** The HDPE cups have to be directed towards the sacroiliac joint to transmit forces perpendicularly from the implant-cement interface

The transmission of load is clearly indicated by the dense bone structure directed from the acetabular roof towards the sacroiliac joint (Fig. 75a). The anchoring structures of a cemented acetabular cup should be inclined such that surfaces which are transmitting load will be perpendicular to these bone structures (Fig. 75b, c). Correctly implanted, the "low profile" design is favourable, because impingement of the femoral component is made impossible. More safety with respect to luxation is achieved by a "high profile" design.

CHAPTER 6
Preparation of the Bone Cement

Cement mixing of PMMA bone cements was carried out in the past with a bowl, a spatula, the powder, and the bottle with monomer (Fig. 76). For the validation every single step of the preparation and application of the bone cement was studied in minor and major research programs and if necessary, the preparation was modified. The polymer powder consists of pearl-like balls ranging from 1 µm to more than 140 µm (Fig. 77). The individual research programs are listed in the ZOW report (1998). The most important findings are presented below.

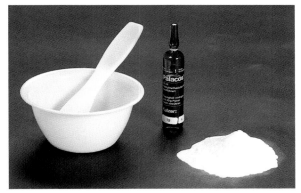

Fig. 76. Bone cement was formerly mixed with a bowl, spatula, powder, and bottle with monomer

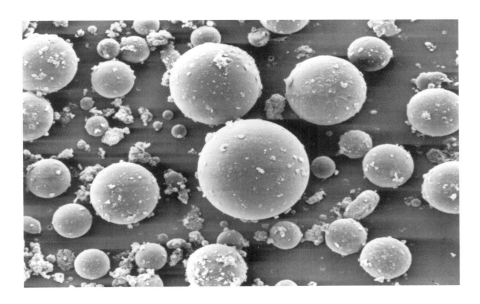

Fig. 77. PMMA polymer powder, SEM

6.1
Advantages of Standard Viscosity Bone Cement

Standard viscosity bone cements are difficult to process at room temperatures. Viscosity can, however, easily be lowered temporarily by storing the bone cement components and the mixing bowl in a refrigerator box at 4°C. In addition, standard viscosity bone cements have a number of advantages which make them superior to the low viscosity group (Table 2).

The low viscosity bone cement might be conflicting with respect to the tolerance of the applicating procedure. This is due to the fact that it is liquid over a long

	Low viscosity bone cement	Standard viscosity bone cement
Fatigue strength	+	++
Tolerance of the procedure	–	+++
Avoidance of intermixing	–	++
Vacuum mixing	+	+++
Pushing aside bone marrow	–	+
Storage at 4°C	–	++
Curve of polymerization	Steep, –	More flat, +++

Table 2. Comparison of low- and standard-viscosity bone cements

period of time and is intermixed very quickly by blood during that time. This becomes apparent when the entire prosthesis component with the bone cement gets pushed out by the restreaming blood due to a hydraulic pressure (Benjamin et al., 1987). The danger with the low-viscosity bone cement is indicated by the steep curve of polymerization. The bone cement remains liquid for a long time and then it hardens quickly. During the steep increase the stem cannot be inserted completely; therefore the processing tolerance is considered as low.

6.2
Cold Storage as a Simple Method To Achieve a Temporarily Lower Viscosity

Standard viscosity bone cements can be cooled from room temperature of 20°–22°C to a component temperature of 1°–4°C in about 6 h if it is taken out of the isolating package. This means that the nurse must store bone cement in a refrigerator (Fig. 78). Temperature measurements in a refrigerator revealed an increase in temperature from bottom to top and front to back. Stable temperatures could only be achieved in a refrigerator box (Fig. 79).

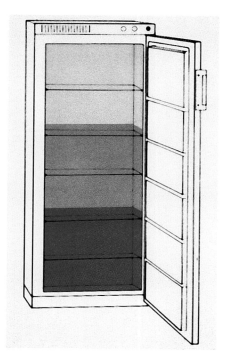

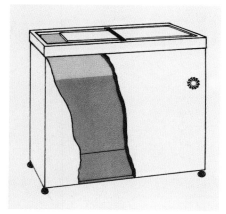

Fig. 79. Refrigerator box achieving stable layering of temperature

Fig. 78. Refrigerator demonstrating different layers of temperature

6.3
Homogeneous and Bubble-Free Mixture

There were no scientific studies reported on the initial mixing. Therefore, a series of studies was necessary in order to demonstrate that the mixture in the way that first the liquid is poured into the container, and then the powder is given into the liquid, is correct (Fig. 80).

The high molecular weight PMMA powder sinks in the liquid, stripping off air bubbles. An even and simultaneous moistening of the polymer spheres occurs faster this way.

In the reverse method, a crust of polymerized material forms under which unmoistened powder is hidden in lumps and causes heterogeneity of the mixture.

The stirrer was not taken into account in any study until recently. Studies showed that the spatula had to be replaced by a Teflon-covered round stirring rod because the spatula would produce large air inclusions which could not be eliminated, even under vacuum conditions; Teflon is advantageous because it does not adhere to bone cement (Fig. 81). The bowl was unfavorable because in the flat monomer lake the polymerization was uneven and perfect homogeneity was not achieved. The best results were found with an Erlenmeyer flask where monomer and powder had better contact because of the higher liquid level due to the diagonal walls of the flask. However, removing the bone cement from the Erlenmeyer flask was difficult. A compromise was found. A cup with a minimum diameter of 55 mm was used in which up to 80 g polymer together with 40 ml monomer could be mixed homogeneously (Fig. 82).

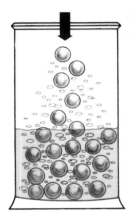

Fig. 80. Polymer is added to the monomer

Fig. 81. Teflon-coated stirrers avoid huge air inclusions

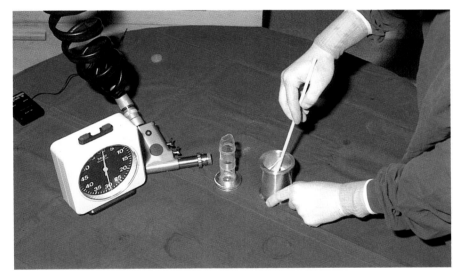

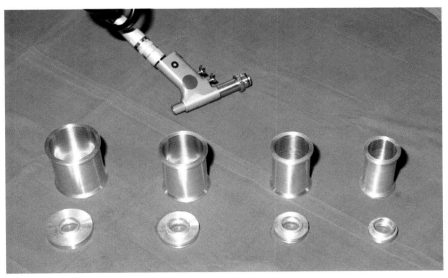

FFig. 82. The mixing bowl must be cylindrical in shape, optimized for a powder mass up to 80 g

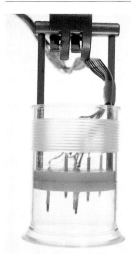

Fig. 83. Three dimensional arrangement of thermal electrodes for determining homogeneity

There was also little literature found about mixing. These studies generally measured only porosity (Haas et al. 1975). Lee et al. (1973) found a decrease in strength dependent more on stirring (revolutions per second) than on the duration of the mixing. Changing the speed of rotation during mixing had not been studied. Eyerer and Jin (1986) concluded that a short mixing time with low speed of stirring gave the best results. Studies of such an approach in our institute resulted in inhomogeneous mixtures. The two parameters, homogeneity and porosity, had to be analyzed separately. The homogeneity was more difficult to measure than the porosity, which was easily accomplished by an image analysis. In our institute, homogeneity was analyzed using a field of thermal electrodes in order to determine the "hot lakes" (monomer) and "cold spots" (polymer). Temperature peaks correspond to the monomer which generates heat wheras polymer conglomerates remain relatively cold (Fig. 83).

Homogeneous mixtures of bone cement indicate polymerization curves with similar paths even at different room temperatures (Fig. 84) Bone cement with fillers (Refobacin Palacos) on the contrary remain heterogeneous even after hours of mixing of antibiotic together with the polymer powder. The heterogeneity is indicated in the polymerization curve (Fig. 85).

Vacuum mixing was first published by Demarest et al. (1983) and introduced into clinical practice by Lidgren et al. (1984). At room temperature vacuum mixing at negative pressures of 150 mbar (0.015 MPa) resulted in boiling of the monomer due to its vapor pressure (Fig. 86) as a function of temperature. Cooled bone cements, however, with components stored at temperatures below 1°–4°C could be mixed bubble-free under these conditions (Figs. 87, 88). Tests concerning the evaporation of monomers showed that after setting the mixture the vapor pressure curve has changed due to the chemical binding of the monomer to the polymer.

It could be concluded from these experiments:

- Standard viscosity bone cement that was stored at 1–4°C could be mixed bubble-free under higher vacuum.
- Low viscosity bone cements could only be mixed under low vacuum conditions (up to 550 mbar = 0.55 MPa).

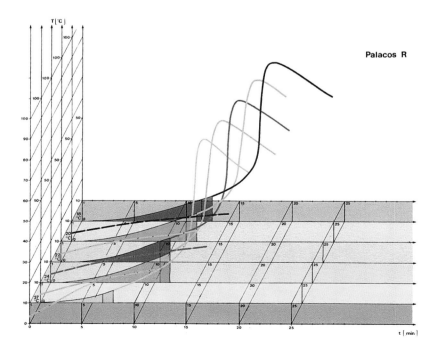

Fig. 84. Polymerization characteristic of Palacos bone cement at different temperatures including body temperature. Triangles, working tolerance

6.3 Homogeneous and Bubble-Free Mixture

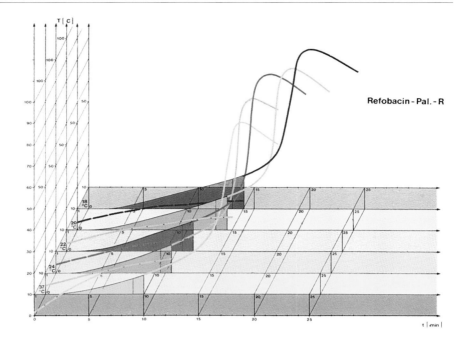

Fig. 85. Polymerization characteristic of Refobacin Palacos revealing in the paths of curves a slight inhomogeneity due to the gentamicin filler

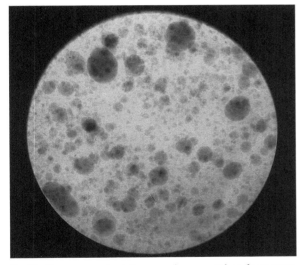

Fig. 86. Bone cement mixing samples were taken from more than 3000 tests (by nurses and physicians). These samples were studied and validated on mammography films. The monomer can be boiled at room temperature under vacuum. Completely bubble-free samples were mixed regularly in nurse training courses

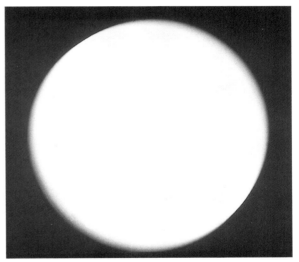

Fig. 87. Cooled standard viscosity bone cements can be mixed bubble free under vacuum

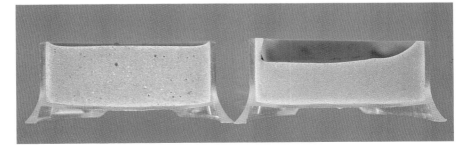

Fig. 88. A comparison of conventionally mixed and vacuum-mixed bone cement, demonstrating that vacuum mixing requires more bone cement to achieve a similar volume

This is not sufficient to completely eliminate the microporosity.
- Vacuum mixing requires more bone cement – vacuum application demands at least 70 g bone cement for the femur and 40 g for the acetabulum

6.4
Prepressurizing Bone Cements, a Conditio Sine Qua Non

Studies of preparations from revision surgeries showed that often the polymer spheres were separated individually from the polymer-monomer compound (Fig. 89). SEM studies of the sphere surfaces demonstrated that there were partly roughened and sometimes completely smooth surfaces (Fig. 90). For clarification, the polymerization process was analyzed in 15-s steps by stopping the chemical process with liquid nitrogen and sublimating the rest of monomers under high vacuum conditions. The frozen stages were air dried, sputtered with gold and documented in the SEM. It could be seen that sometimes only 30%–40% of the polymer bead surfaces were moistened with monomer (Figs. 91, 92). On the other hand, a 100% contact could be achieved with application of pressure between 3 and 4 bar ($3–4 \cdot 10^5$ Pa). The same was found for fillers as zirconium dioxide, barium sulfate, gentamicin, tricalcium phosphate and hydroxyapatite. Test series with standard "three point bending" tests showed that more than 85% of the total bending strength after 1 min of prepressurization could be achieved.

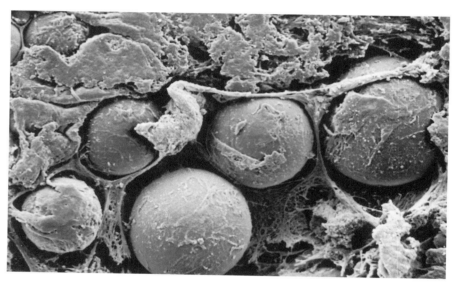

Fig. 89. Sample of bone cement taken out during revision 7 years after the operation, revealing bone cement adjacent to the metal. The polymer spheres are freed by ingrown fibroblasts (SEM)

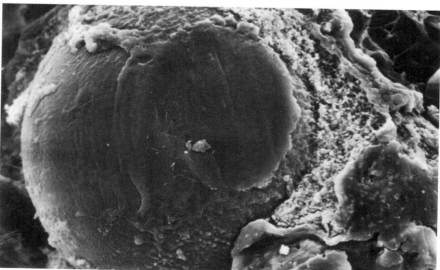

Fig. 90. Embedded polymer bead. The surface is partly smooth and partly chemically etched by the monomer

6.4 Prepressurizing Bone Cements, a Conditio Sine Qua Non

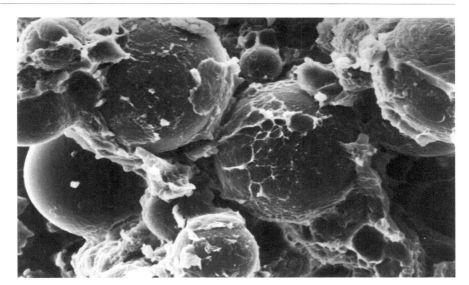

Fig. 91. Status of polymerization 15 s after setting the mixture of polymer and monomer; some of the beads did not come into contact with the monomer (SEM)

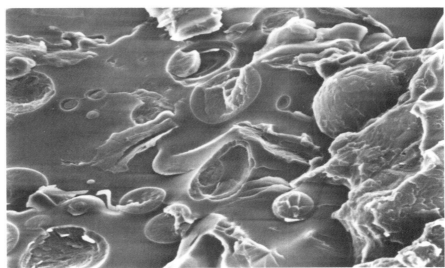

Fig. 92. Fracture sample of hardened bone cement. Many beads are not fully embedded in the secondarily polymerizing matrix (SEM)

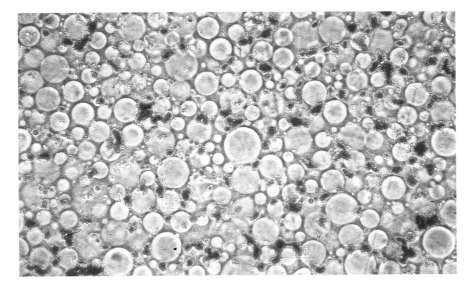

Fig. 93. Thin cross-section of prepressurized and vacuum-mixed bone cement in the phase contrast microscope. The dense line around all beads indicates a 100% contact with the secondarily polymerized matrix

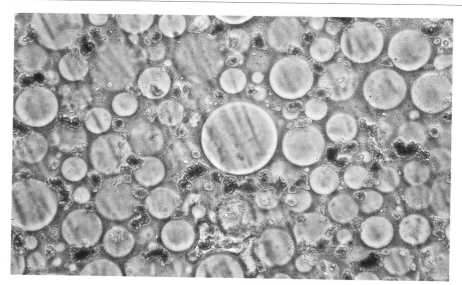

Fig. 94. Sample which is prepressurized but not vacuum-mixed. The embedded air bubble has been deformed

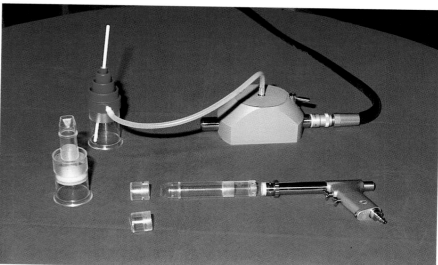

Fig. 95. Complete equipment for vacuum mixing and prepressurizing bone cements. Vacuum pump, validated disposable systems and cement gun

The best demonstration of the interface between polymer and monomer can be given in phase contrast. The samples, which were mixed under vacuum and prepressurized, show an increased strength of 20%–30% during fatigue tests (Soltesz and Ege 1992; Fig. 93). Keller and Lautenschlager (1983) achieved the highest density with a pressure increase of 13.8 MPa during the entire hardening phase. The authors described the samples as almost porous-free. In addition, they observed a regular morphological structure of the matrix and thus concluded that improved binding between polymer spheres and matrix had occurred. Under clinical condition only for a limited time span pressure can be applied on the polymerizing bone cement.

We can conclude from these experiments that prepressurization is a conditio sine qua non for all kind of

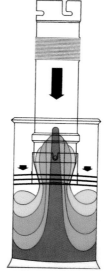

Fig. 96. Extruding bone cement avoids an effect of body temperature and contact with gloves which are permeable for monomer

bone cements in order to achieve a 100% binding of the PMMA components. It takes care of a 100% embedding of all beads and fillers which has a tremendous impact on fatigue life. Prepressurization does not eliminate air bubbles (Fig. 94); it deforms them. The mechanical energy applied to the bone cement mass shortens its polymerization time by about 1 min. Vacuum mixing and prepressurization are considered as optimal (Fig. 95); hand contact must be avoided (Fig. 96).

6.5
Application of the Bubble-Free Bone Cement

A retrograde filling is widely used for the application of bubble-free bone cement. Using the nozzle, the analysis with colored cement portions showed, however, characteristics of turbulences during the application of bone cement in the laboratory (Fig. 97). Filling the model by motorized syringe through a nozzle took 21 s, not including the delivery of bone cement from the nozzle itself; the later process took another 34 s. In addition, the lamination of the cement mass could not be avoided. Studies with the nozzle using the Benjamin et al. model (1987) revealed blood, debris and air inclusions between the laminations (Fig. 98). In comparison to that, the vacuum application, using the same model, showed two essential differences: (a) vacuum application led to complete and artifact-free filling of the bony bed in about

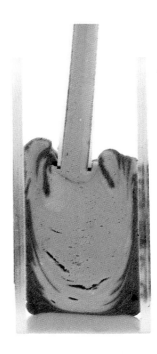

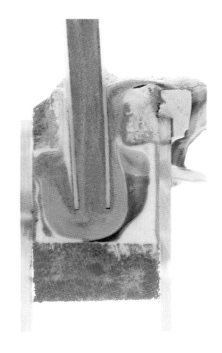

Fig. 97. A retrograde filling using a nozzle produces substantial turbulence, including air, blood, and debris

Fig. 98. A study based on the Benjamin et al. model (1987) reveals the inclusion of blood into the cement mass

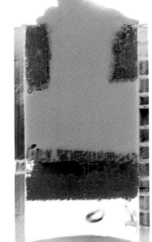

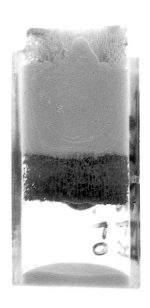

Fig. 99. Workshop model demonstrating the artifact free filling into the bony bed within 1.5 s

Fig. 100. Workshop model after conventional retrograde filling using a nozzle reveals multiple laminations; time for filling was 21 s

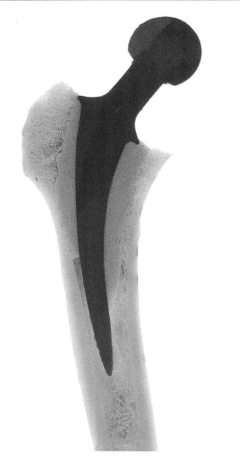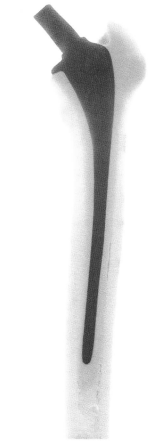

Fig. 101. Incomplete filling of a human dry bone at room temperature with a standard viscosity, conventionally mixed bone cement

Fig. 102. Vacuum-mixed and vacuum-applied bone cement using a standard viscosity bone cement and a long stem; artifact-free and complete filling resulted within 2 s

1–2 s; (b) the cement was suctioned bubble free into the dry bony bed (Figs. 99, 100).

Artefact-free cement filling cannot be achieved using retrograde filling with a nozzle, even under favorable laboratory conditions.

This was confirmed in practical workshops on human bone comparing the nozzle and vacuum techniques. For this purpose, cadaver bones were corroded, defattened and treated with 5% H_2O_2 and dried. The surgeons could test different stems and procedures. The stems used were replicas made from plastic which were easy to cut after the exercise. The cut samples were polished, dried and then sent to the surgeon. Incomplete filling resulted after conventional procedures in most cases (Fig. 101) while vacuum application yielded an artifact-free filling even with long stems (Fig. 102).

CHAPTER 7
Preparation of the Femur

7.1 Opening of the Medullary Canal and Implantation Axis

Charnley (1979) reached the entrance to the medullary canal through his trochanteric osteotomy. Müller, with his "Setzholz" prosthesis (Müller and Ellmiger 1979), used a direct lateral approach through the bone of the greater trochanter. With his straight stem he standardized this lateral approach and used it for the construction of his self-locking straight stem. He could overcome the problem of varization with this new procedure.

The same direct access is practised by all traumatologists during intramedullary nailing of the femur.

If one overlays a cross-section of the distal femoral tube (17–21 cm below) to the trochanteric plane (Fig. 103), which is the cross section of the plane where the femoral neck passes over to the bone of the greater trochanter, the medullary canal can be reached through the projected canal in a straight way. This point is called "knee of the greater trochanter."

The medullary canal is opened with an 11.2 mm diamond cutting tool in the knee of the greater trochanter.

In the axial view it is quite obvious that the posterior wall of the neck is in straight alignment to the posterior wall of the diaphyseal tube; the diamond is inserted within the neck along the posterior wall of the neck. This line is the posterior tangential alignment (pta) (Fig. 104). The diamond tool (Fig. 105) is used at full speed (800–1000 rpm) in combination with an inner rinsing solution at a pressure of 0.05 MPa (500 mbar).

In case that the free medullary canal was not met during the first attempt and the bone cylinder adheres to the femoral cortex an elongated extractor is inserted by gentle blows of a plastic hammer; the bone cylinder is then twisted off and pushed out of the extractor in a retrograde manner.

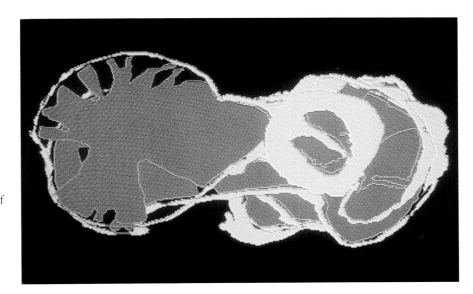

Fig. 103. The cross-section of the midshaft femur is overlain upon the plane of the greater trochanter and thus indicates the point through which the medullary canal can be reached in a straight way

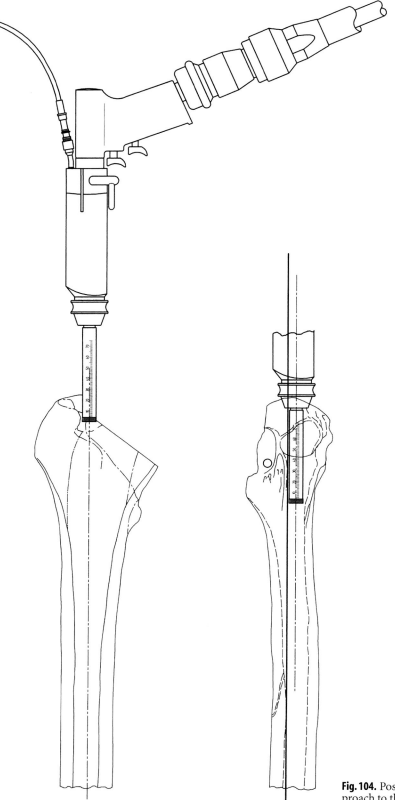

Fig. 104. Posterior tangential alignment and approach to the medullary canal using the straight diamond tool

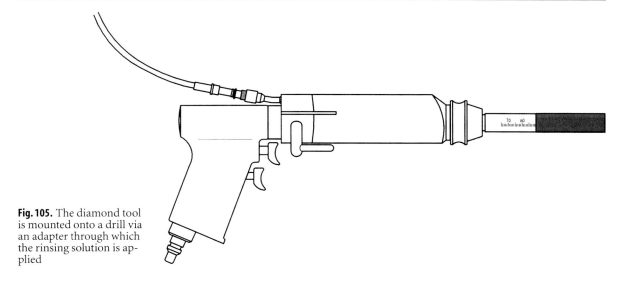

Fig. 105. The diamond tool is mounted onto a drill via an adapter through which the rinsing solution is applied

7.2
Surgical Diamond Instrumentation

In any histological laboratory processing nondemineralized tissue a diamond technique is considered the method of choice to process bone. Sharp instruments and rasps destroy and break bone, oscillating saws burn and fracture it. The wet grinding process using diamonds (Fig. 106) does not traumatize bone. The only artefact found histologically was a slight demineralization up to a depth of 30 µm due to the washing solution. This was concluded from staining of bone samples with basic fuchsin which stains bone less mineralized than 80% (Fig. 107). The cells adjacent to the cutting line were vital, stained and contained a normal nucleus (Draenert and Draenert 1987).

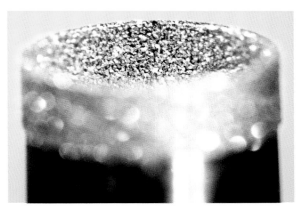

Fig. 106. High-precision diamond-coated tool

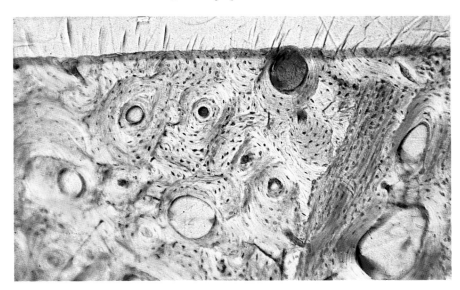

Fig. 107. Bone biopsy taken from human femoral cortex stained with basic fuchsin reveals slight demineralization as the only artefact

In a study in which 8 different cutter heads were compared (Fig. 108) the diamond had the best results. The wet-grinding procedure (Fig. 109) remains after all experiments the method of choice to prepare the bony bed of the stem. Diamond tools coated broadly along the outside of the cylinder (Fig. 110) cover all needs for preparation of the bony bed; with long tubes dysplastic femurs can be prepared through the canal isthmus of the diaphysis.

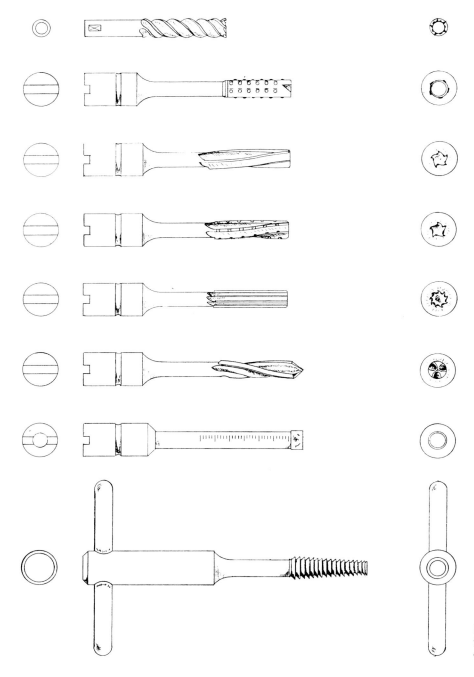

Fig. 108. Eight different cutter heads compared in a study on animal bone

7.2 Surgical Diamond Instrumentation

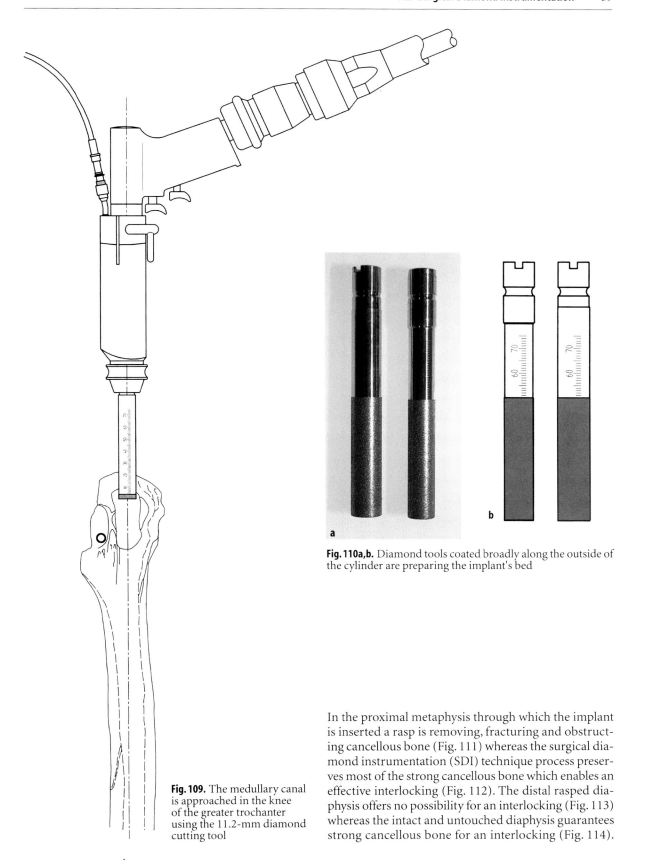

Fig. 109. The medullary canal is approached in the knee of the greater trochanter using the 11.2-mm diamond cutting tool

Fig. 110a,b. Diamond tools coated broadly along the outside of the cylinder are preparing the implant's bed

In the proximal metaphysis through which the implant is inserted a rasp is removing, fracturing and obstructing cancellous bone (Fig. 111) whereas the surgical diamond instrumentation (SDI) technique process preserves most of the strong cancellous bone which enables an effective interlocking (Fig. 112). The distal rasped diaphysis offers no possibility for an interlocking (Fig. 113) whereas the intact and untouched diaphysis guarantees strong cancellous bone for an interlocking (Fig. 114).

Chapter 7 Preparation of the Femur

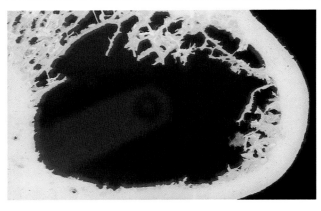

Fig. 111. Cross-section of the proximal metaphysis of a femur after rasping the implant's bed

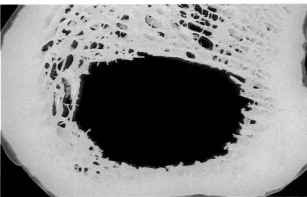

Fig. 112. Cross-section after use of the diamond technique. The strong cancellous bone must be preserved

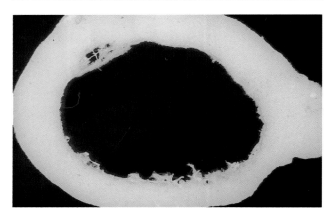

Fig. 113. Rasping the diaphysis means removing all bone structures for interlocking

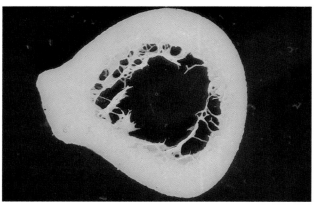

Fig. 114. For cementing femoral stems it is a conditio sine qua non not to touch it by a rasp. The strong cancellous bone must be preserved, as shown here in a femur of a 58-year-old man

7.3
Drainage of the Medullary Canal

The drill jig is introduced into the open canal (11.2 mm) without applying any force (Fig. 115). The jig is calibrated at the transition of the femoral neck to the greater trochanter.

If the jig cannot be introduced easily the diamond-coated drill is used to grind first to the lateral side parallel to the canal axis (Fig. 116a) and then gently towards the posterior wall of the femoral neck (Fig. 116b). With the jig in position it is rotated from the exact lateral position 15° anteriorly: through a skin incision (2.0 cm) the trocar is introduced using the hammer, first, to hit the trocar and second, to hit the sharp drill guide onto the bone. In this way, the traumatization of the periosteum by the drill is avoided; the 4.5 mm drill which is thickened in its middle portion does not allow any play within the tube and is cutting only one cortex. The cannula is screwed in while the guide is pressed to the bone.

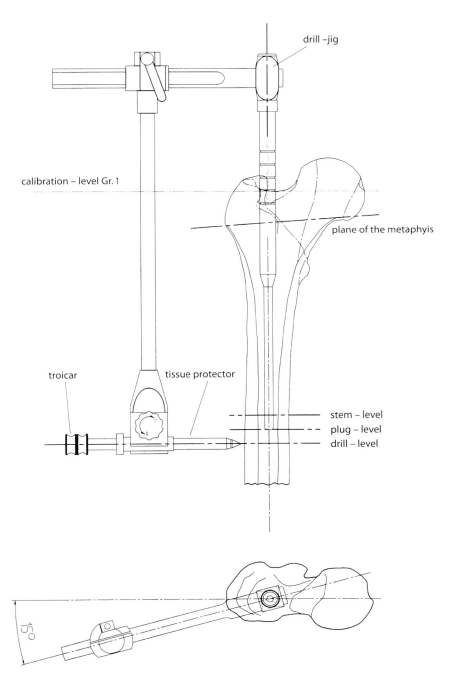

Fig. 115. The jig is introduced without any force

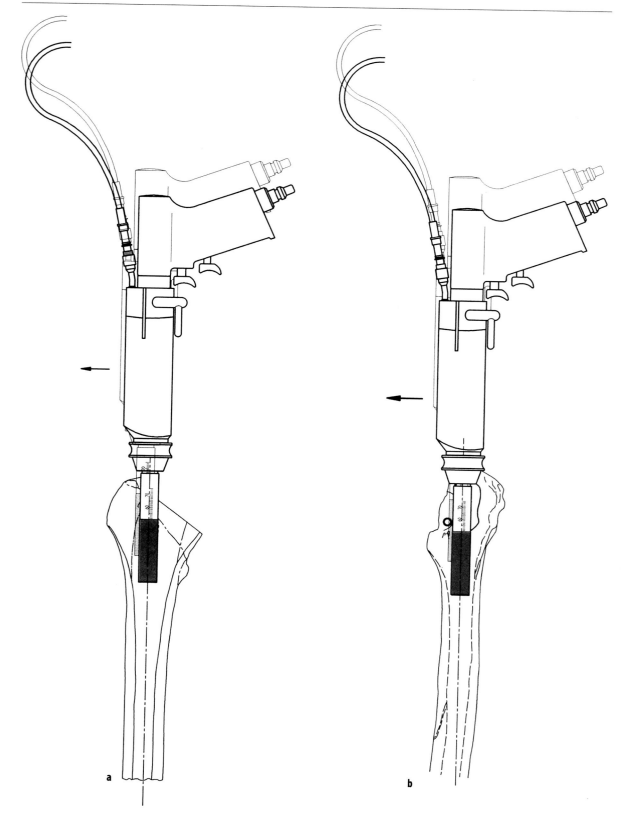

Fig. 116a,b. Widening of the channel by parallel grinding laterally and posteriorly is needed if no free access has been achieved

There are two calibration marks: the first indicates that the tip of the cannula appears in the femoral canal and the second that its tip has reached the center of the cavity (Fig. 117). In this position the cannula remains till the plug is placed.

The jig is now removed and the same drill is used to prepare the seat for the proximal cannula. This cannula is needed to drain blood and fat during insertion of the cement and during placement of the implant. This works efficiently and unaffected by cement. The drill hole is exactly placed in the fovea intertrochanterica (Fig. 118). The hole is drilled parallel to the posterior wall of the neck up to a depth of 1–2 cm. Having the screw placed, the lumen is freed from any debris or coagle using the tappet (2.8 mm). With the drill mounted, Adam's arch is tunneled with two 4.5-mm drill holes perpendicular to the neck and parallel to the osteotomy. This is necessary according to the anatomical structure of the funnel-shaped cancellous bone the honeycombs of which cannot be filled up with bone cement except through a tunnel which gives access to the scaffolding of the medial support radially, circularly and in axial direction.

The cannulated screw is protected by intact cancellous bone from obstruction (Fig. 119). Since the ascending branch of the nutrient artery is found in the posterior scaffolding of metaphyseal cancellous bone mainly light red arterial blood is suctioned through this cannula (Fig. 120). Any increase in pressure in the medullary canal is discharged through the distal and proximal cannula. Through the two cannulae twice 20 ml Ringer's solution are injected and then the vacuum pumps are connected.

Fig. 117. The cannula is screwed in until the second calibration mark disappears

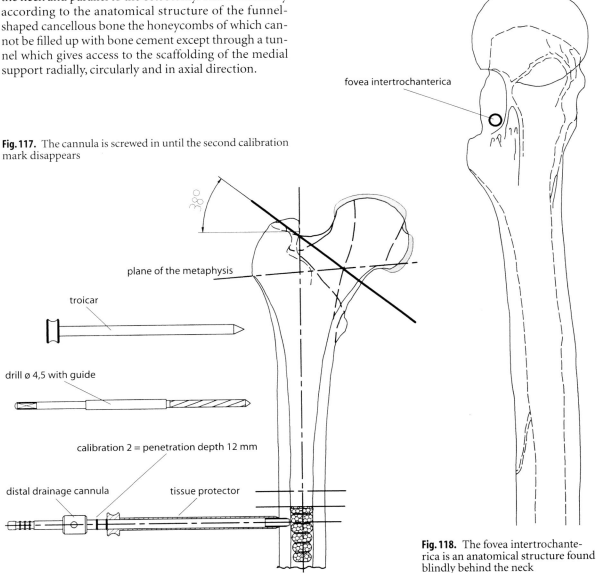

Fig. 118. The fovea intertrochanterica is an anatomical structure found blindly behind the neck

Chapter 7 Preparation of the Femur

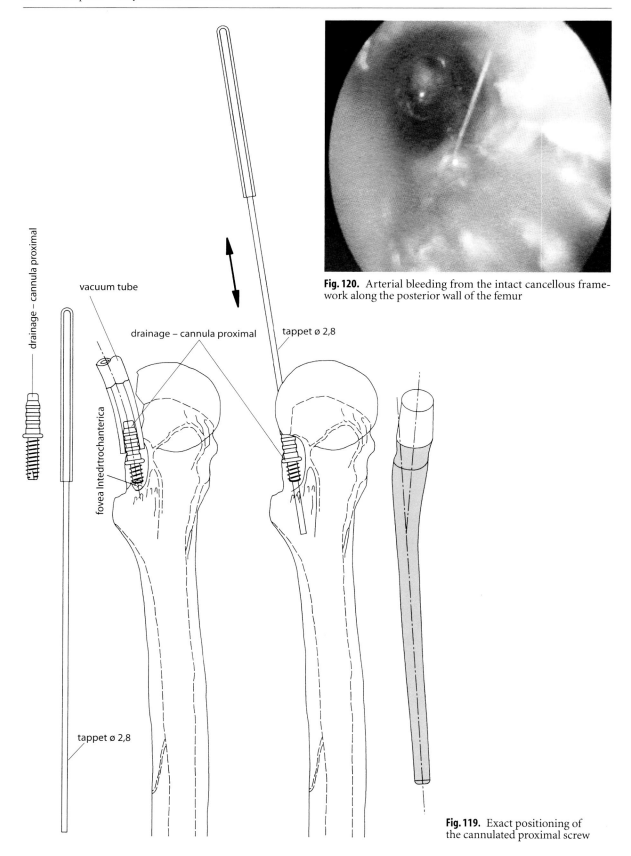

Fig. 120. Arterial bleeding from the intact cancellous framework along the posterior wall of the femur

Fig. 119. Exact positioning of the cannulated proximal screw

7.4
Preparation of the Implant's Bed

After placement of the cannulae the bed is prepared using the diamond-coated grinder. Beginning in the depth of the canal, side pressure is only applied during retraction of the drilling machine; in this way a smoothly ground surface is prepared without any steps. This is done in all directions, laterally and medially (Fig. 121a) and anteriorly and posteriorly (Fig. 121b).

To prepare the bed for the stem's shoulder the cancellous bone in the greater trochanter is ground behind

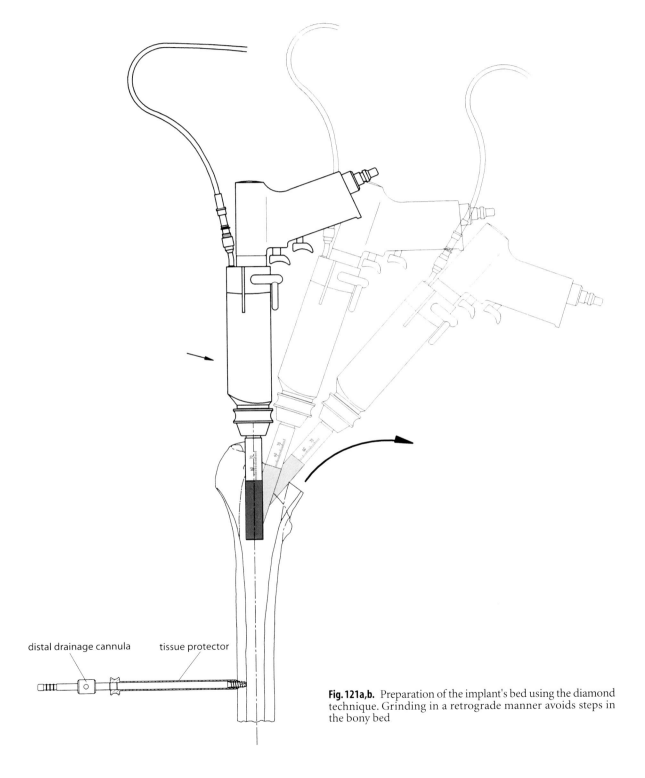

Fig. 121a,b. Preparation of the implant's bed using the diamond technique. Grinding in a retrograde manner avoids steps in the bony bed

the line to the opening canal. The trial stem is now placed and reposition with a trial head is performed. Luxation tendency under tension and different positions of flexion and adduction is checked (Fig. 122).

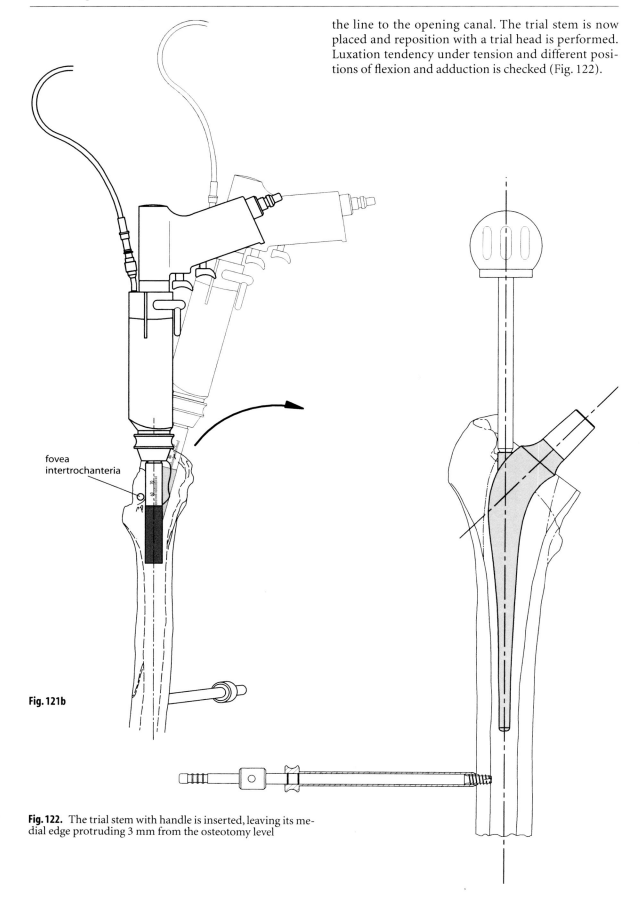

fovea intertrochanteria

Fig. 121b

Fig. 122. The trial stem with handle is inserted, leaving its medial edge protruding 3 mm from the osteotomy level

7.5
Lavage

The primary stability was determined by the degree of intertrabecular interlocking of the prosthesis component; the interlocking was achieved by bone cement. The penetration depth of bone cement was described as a function of viscosity and applied pressure (Markolf and Amstutz 1976; Halawa et al. 1978; Krause et al. 1982) The medullary cavity plug was implanted with the low viscosity bone cement (Amstutz et al. 1976), and the spongiosa medullary cavities had to be cleaned with a brush and pressure lavage (Miller and Serot 1978; Lee and Ling 1981; Sherman et al. 1983).

High-pressure jet lavage itself can push out bone marrow emboli (Clarius 1996). The lavage using Ringer solution containing 3%–5% H_2O_2 must start gently, washing out the fat marrow first, over the whole length of the stem. After removal of the fat the pressure is increased till the cancellous bone appears white and clean. No part of the bony bed should be forgotten (Fig. 123). Cancellous bone not cleaned cannot be filled with bone cement.

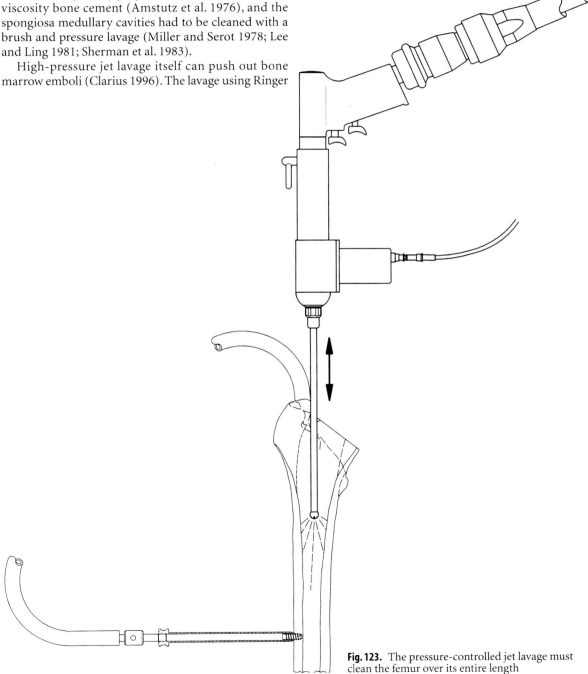

Fig. 123. The pressure-controlled jet lavage must clean the femur over its entire length

7.6
Plugging the Medullary Cavity

The medullary cavity plug is a development that started to be used in clinical practice due to the low viscosity bone cement invention (Amstutz et al. 1976; Oh et al. 1978). The plug hinders the entrance of cement into the depths of the medullary canal and it results in significantly improved interlocking (Markolf and Amstutz 1976).

It performs another essential function during the drainage of the distal drill hole:

The medullary cavity plug must hinder bone cement from entering the drill hole and the drainage cannula.

The medullary canal is typically conformed in its different compartments. The medullary cavity above the canal isthmus is oval in shape with its large diameter in the sagittal direction. A cylindrical implant cannot plug the cavity. If, however, the strong cancellous bone along the cortex is not removed, a well-shaped stopper (Fig. 124) will close the lumen for bone cement by elastically deforming the spongiosa.

After washing of the implant's bed the canal's isthmus is measured. Allowing a tolerance of 1 mm, four different balls on the measuring instrument correspond to eight different sizes of stoppers (Fig. 125).

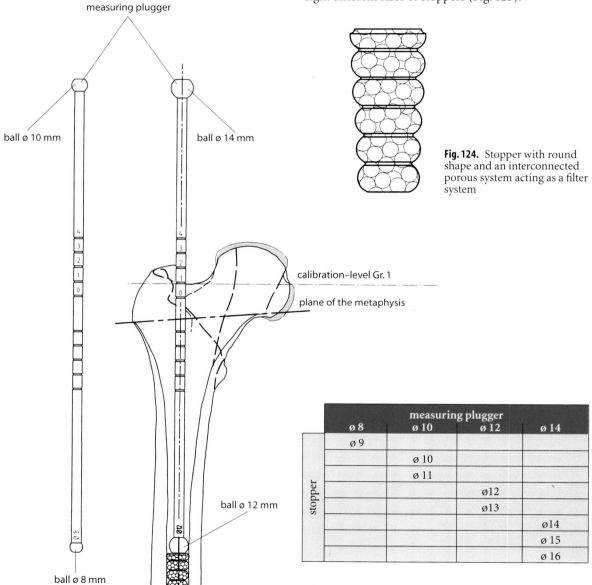

Fig. 124. Stopper with round shape and an interconnected porous system acting as a filter system

stopper	measuring plugger			
	ø 8	ø 10	ø 12	ø 14
	ø 9			
		ø 10		
		ø 11		
			ø 12	
			ø 13	
				ø 14
				ø 15
				ø 16

Fig. 125. A combined instrument with two different diameter balls is used for measuring the canal's isthmus

The plug for the vacuum technique consists of a completely interconnecting porosity (Fig. 124), it acts as a filter for the vacuum cannula (Draenert 1989). The plug is plunged into the heparin-Ringer solution and then mounted to a flexible rod and inserted into the canal along its axis (Fig. 126). No hammer should be used together with the applicator. As soon as the applicator is caught, the clamps must be released and the instrument retracted; the corresponding plugger is now introduced, the distal cannula is screwed out till the first calibration mark appears again at the drill guide, a K-wire is introduced and then the plug is forwarded till the K-wire has been reached. After removal of the K-wire, the plug is carefully placed 1 cm below the stem's tip, looking carefully onto the calibration mark.

The medullary cavity plug ensures that the vacuum fully develops, and that the cannula is not obstructed; coagulation of blood in the plug should be avoided using heparin. Therefore the medullary cavity plug is dipped into a heparinized Ringer solution before its application (10,000 IU heparin in 300 ml Ringer solution). A high pore volume must be provided which can take up bone cement.

The plug must be conical in shape so that it cannot pass the cannula which is first screwed forward touching the stopper and then twisted back one-fourth of a revolution. Its exterior contour must be rounded, so that it does not become hooked or blocked.

In the case of revision an acrylate plug provides a tight bond to the bone cement which is suctioned in. The stopper is removed with the titanium scissel heated by ultrasound.

After the plug is placed, the femoral canal is sealed with two pads soaked with 5% H_2O_2.

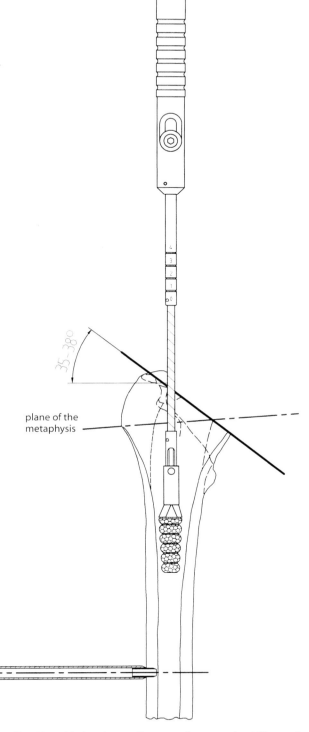

Fig. 126. With the plug applicator, no hammer should be used

7.7
Heparinization, Cementation, and Implantation

After preparation of the medullary canal the coagulation of blood is avoided, by injecting twice 20 ml of a heparin-Ringer solution through the two cannulae; 300 ml Ringer's solution containing 10,000 IU heparin. The vacuum pump is not shut off but slowed down to half the pressure, and the bone cement is ordered. Standard viscosity bone cement is preferred.

Setting the bone cement mix going by adding the powder to the liquid, all components cooled down to 4°C are mixed under vacuum and prepressurized.

During prepressurization for at least 1 min twice 20 ml of the above heparin Ringer solution is injected into the medullary canal. The pads are removed and the seal is mounted with the cartridge into the open femoral end (Fig. 127); full vacuum is now applied and after 2 s the bone cement is injected. From that time, the medullary canal is discharged by vacuum through the two cannulae.

The lateral wall of the seal is now incised (Fig. 128) and the stem is introduced holding the seal firmly in its position thus avoiding that bone cement can escape.

The seal's cylindrical part is used to find the correct axial orientation and access to the medullary canal for the stem. During insertion of the last third of the stem the lateral part of the seal is opened and only medially firmly fixed till the stem is completely placed by hand; now the seal is removed and overflowing bone cement is taken off flush to the osteotomy surface using a spatula. The stem should be left unattached (Fig. 129), vacuum is reduced to half and in case of obstruction of the proximal cannula the 2.8-mm plugger is pushed through until arterial blood is again clearly visible in the silicon tube.

After hardening of the cement, indicated by a cement ball which is formed and held in the nurse's hand taken from remaining bone cement in the bowl, the cone protector is removed and the cone carefully cleaned. The definitive ball is fixed and the leg repositioned using the lever arm of the repositioning instrument; a forced pull to the leg should be avoided.

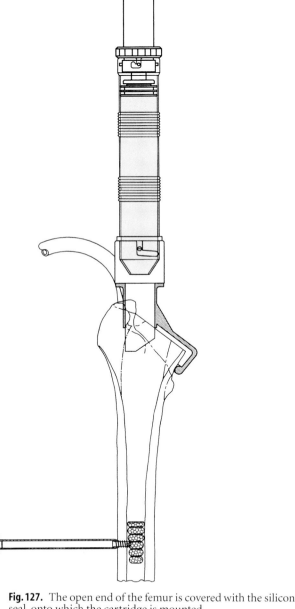

Fig. 127. The open end of the femur is covered with the silicon seal, onto which the cartridge is mounted

7.7 Heparinization, Cementation, and Implantation

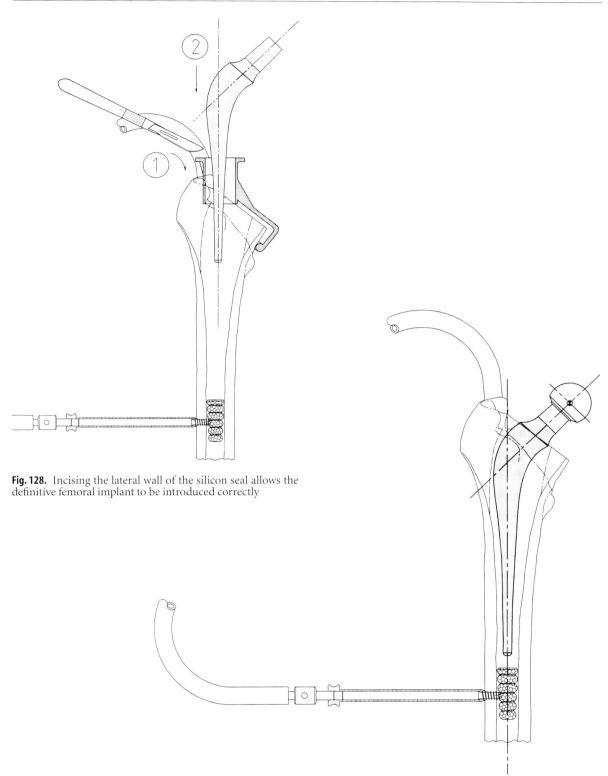

Fig. 128. Incising the lateral wall of the silicon seal allows the definitive femoral implant to be introduced correctly

Fig. 129. Insertion of the definitive implant. There is no need to hold the implant during polymerization of bone cement with the vacuum technique

CHAPTER 8

Scientific Background of Vacuum Application

8.1
The Problem of Thromboembolism and Drainage of the Medullary Canal

Pulmonary embolism (Table 3) and deep vein thromboses (Table 4) are the most common complications associated with artificial hip joint replacements procedures.

Studies by Breed (1974), Kallos et al. (1974), Schlag (1974), Schlag et al. (1976), Ulrich et al. (1986), and Draenert and Ulrich (1989) have explained the relationship of intramedullary pressure increase and thromboembolic complications. Transesophageal echocardiography (TEE) is considered the method of choice to identify bone marrow embolisms of the medullary cavity intraoperatively. Although the relationship is known the complication rate has insignificantly decreased (Tables 4, 5). One can presume that the studies by Patterson et al. (1991) and Bogner and Landauer (1991) address embolisms out of the medullary canal, thus bone marrow embolisms.

The increase in the intramedullary pressure during insertion of the stem is documented in Table 5; clinical fatal events (Table 6) and results from applied research (Table 5) underline the importance of these values for the understanding of the etiology.

The Zentrum für Orthopädische Wissenschaften in Munich conducted a multicenter study at three German clinics in which patients who had undergone an artificial hip joint replacement were observed intraoperatively by means of two-dimensional TEE echocardiography. In order to analyze cardiovascular reaction during THR procedures the end expiratory pCO_2 and the arterial pO_2 were measured. All together 95 patients were monitored using TEE during the entire operation and the resulting videos were evaluated by Clarius (1996; Table 7). All manipulations that showed embolization out of the medullary canal were recorded; 29.8% of the

Table 3. Pulmonary embolism with artificial hip joint replacement

Reference	n	Incidence (%)	Diagnostic method	Fatalincidence (%)
Daniel et al. (1972)	242	2.1	Thorax X-ray	0.4
Sevitt (1972)	112	NR	NR	5.4
Johnson et al. (1977)	7959	7.9	Clinical	1.0
without prophylaxis	1174	15.2	Clinical	2.3
Tscherne et al. (1978)	323	4.3	Lung scintigraphy	0.3
Dorr et al. (1979)	25	6.0	Lung scintigraphy	NR
Fredin and Nillius (1982)	1324	NR	Clinical	0.7
Modig et al. (1983)	30	33.0	Lung scintigraphy	NR
Harris et al. (1984)	73	19.0	Lung scintigraphy	NR
Liedloff et al. (1984)	200	7.0	Clinical	1.5
Kakkar et al. (1985)	500	0.6	Clinical	0.2
Montrey et al. (1985)	248	9.5	Lung scintigraphy	NR
Fredin and Rosberg (1986)	51	23.2	Lung scintigraphy	NR
Siebler et al. (1988)	282	NR	Clinical	2.8
Seelig et al. (1989)	689	0.9	Clinical	0.3
Wille-Jörgensen et al. (1989)	65	9.0	Lung scintigraphy	NR
Zippel (1990)	2000	1.9	Clinical	0.7
Pellegrini et al. (1996)	347	0.3	Clinical	NR
Clarke et al. (1997)	104	1.0	Clinical	NR

Table 4. Deep leg vein thrombosis with artificial hip joint replacement

Reference	n	Incidence (%)	Diagnostic method	Medical prevention
Evarts and Feil (1971)	56	54	Phlebography	No
	50	14	Phlebography	Yes
Stamatakis et al. (1976)	52	54	Phlebography	NR
Stamatakis et al. (1977)	160	51	Phlebography	NR
Johnson et al. (1978)	50	54	Phlebography	Yes
Tscherne et al. (1978)	323	42	Radio-phlebog.	Yes
Kakkar et al. (1979)	182	21	Radio-phlebog.	Yes
Nillius and Nylander (1979)	134	58	Phlebography	Yes
Thorburn et al. (1980)	47	54	Phlebography	No
Modig et al. (1983)	30	77	Phlebography	No
Nilsen et al. (1984)	22	59	Phlebography	No
Kakkar et al. (1985)	500	26	Phlebography	Yes
Francis et al. (1986)	13	31	Phlebography	Yes
Fredin and Rosberg (1986)	51	45	Phlebography	Yes
Beisaw et al. (1988)	78	52	Radio-phlebog.	No
	78	25	Radio-phlebog.	Yes
Davis et al. (1988)	140	27	Radio-fibrin.	Yes
Borris et al. (1989)	60	46	Phlebography	NR
Liedloff and Brauckhoff (1989)	200	28	Radio-phlebog.	Yes
Lotke et al. (1996)	133	16	Phlebography	Yes
Pellegrini et al. (1996)	347	23	Phlebography	Yes
Clarke et al. (1997)	104	32	Phlebography	No
Eriksson et al (1997)	351	7 (desirudin) 23 (heparin)	Phlebography	Yes

Table 5. Intramedullary pressure during implantation of the stem

Reference	Intramedullary pressure (mmHg)		Method
	Without drill hole	With distal drill hole	
Ohnsorge (1971)	3460	1990	Femur
Phillips et al. (1973)	1900	–	Intraoperative
Breed (1974)	868	100	Animal experiment
Hallin (1974)	680	–	Intraoperative
Kallos et al. (1974)	900	250	Animal experiment
Tronzo et al. (1974)	575	–	Intraoperative
Von Issendorff and Ritter (1977)	3830	736	Femur
Indong et al. (1978)	9750	–	Femur
Drinker et al. (1981)	9450	–	Animal experiment
Engsaeter et al. (1984)	583	35	Intraoperative
Orsini et al. (1987)	1700	–	Animal experiment
Wenda et al. (1988)	1140	140	Intraoperative
Elmaraghy et al. (1998)	325 (reaming), 109 (lavage), 449 (cementing), 432 (l. + c.)	–	Animal experiment

Table 6. Publications concerning intraoperative complications with artificial hip joint replacement

Reference	Diagnosis	Cardiac arrest syndrome (n=70)	Deaths (n=46)	Autopsies (n=18)	Cause of death
Burgess (1970)	SHF	1	1	1	Fat embolism
Charnley (1970b)	NR	4	2		NR
Hyland and Robins (1970)	SHF	1	1	1	Air and fat embolism
Powell et al. (1970)	SHF	3	0		
Cohen and Smith (1971)	TEP-We.	1	1	1	Fat and bone marrow embolism
Dandy (1971)	SHF	4	2	2	Fat embolism
Gresham et al. (1971)	SHF	2	2	2	Fat embolism
Michelinakis et al. (1971)	SHF	2	0		
Phillips et al. (1971)	SHF	1	1	1	Fat and bone marrow embolism
Schulitz et al. (1971)	CA	3	2	1	Fat embolism
Thomas et al. (1971)	SHF	1	1		NR
Kepes et al. (1972)	SHF	2	2	1	Bone marrow embolism
Newens and Volz (1972)	SHF	1	0		
Peebles et al. (1972)	SHF	1	1		NR
Sevitt (1972)	SHF	2	2	2	Fat embolism
DeAngelis and Kenneth (1973)	TEP-We., CA	2	0		
Milne (1973)	CA	1	0		
Nice (1973)	SHF	1	1		NR
Tronzo et al.. (1974)	NR	1	1		NR
Jones (1975)	NR	1	1		Fat embolism
Hyderally and Miller (1976)	Path. SHF	1	1		NR
Beckenbaugh and Ilstrup (1978)	NR	1	1		NR
Engsæter et al. (1984)	NR	1	1	1	Fat embolism
Hochmeister et al. (1987)	SHF	1	1	1	Fat and bone marrow embolism
Zichner (1987)	NR	10	3		NR
Maxeiner (1988)	SHF	3	3	1	Fat embolism
Egbert et al. (1989)	Path. SHF	1	1	1	Fat and bone marrow embolism
Bogner and Landauer (1991)	SHF	10	10	1	No sign of embolism
Patterson et al. (1991)	SHF	10	10	1	No sign of embolism

Table 7. Confirmed embolism with total endoprosthesis surgeries of the hip (from Clarius 1996)

Time	n	Patients with embolism				Embolism size (cm²)						Total emboli	
		n	%	n >0.5	%	<0.5	1	≤1.5	≤2	≤2.5	>2.5	>0 cm²	>0.5 cm²
Double cup prep.	95	11	11.6	3	3.2	17	2	1	0	0	0	20	3
Double cup jet lavage	14	1	7.1	1	7.1	1	1	0	0	0	0	2	1
Double cup test	94	1	1.1	1	1.1	1	3	0	1	0	0	5	4
Double cup implant.	94	28	29.8	16	17.0	27	9	7	6	2	4	55	28
Shifting	94	9	9.6	5	5.3	8	4	2	0	1	0	15	7
Shaft preparation	94	13	13.8	8	8.5	8	8	1	1	0	0	18	10
Plug insertion	90	1	1.1	1	1.1	1	1	0	0	0	0	2	1
Test reposition	94	3	3.2	3	3.2	2	1	1	1	1	0	6	4
Shaft implantation	94	68	72.3	47	50.0	106	66	30	8	6	5	221	115
Reposition	94	66	70.2	52	55.3	80	66	21	9	2	8	186	106

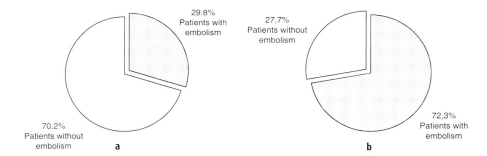

Fig. 130. a Emboli are shown by TEE in 29.8% of all cup implantations (Clarius 1996).
b TEE registers events in 72.3% of all femoral implants (Clarius 1996)

patients showed emboli during cup implantation (Fig. 130), and in 72.3% of the shaft implantations up to 5 cm large emboli were documented. It was surprising that in 70.2% of the cases embolization out of the medullary canal was recorded during repositioning of leg. The latter could not be avoided by the vacuum technique. It proved that during rasping of the medullary canal preformed emboli were formed in the draining veins along the linea aspera. The linea aspera can be considered the venous drainage of the femur along its entire length, as was demonstrated in femoral neck fractures (Fig. 131) and in a laboratory experiment; the medullary cavity content was cleared along the linea aspera in the laboratory experiment in which a vacuum environment was applied to the whole femur (Fig. 132).

A second clinical study was performed by the Zentrum für Orthopädische Wissenschaften at the University of Erlangen considering the "diamond technique"

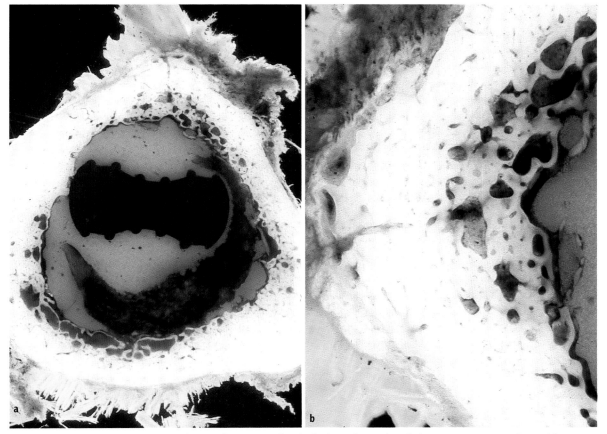

Fig. 131. a Cross-section of a human femur of a patient who died after a femoral neck fracture was operated on with a THR. The medullary canal is filled in all draining veins through the linea aspera with coagulated blood. **b** Linea aspera of the same cross-section revealing an embolus ready for shot

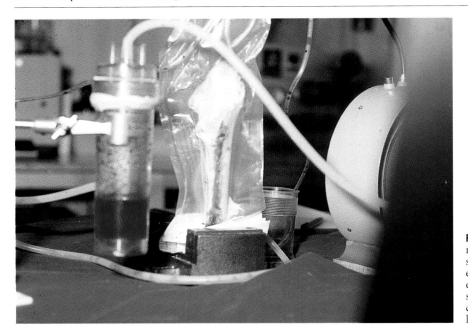

Fig. 132. Drainage of the medullary cavity is demonstrated in a simple laboratory experiment. A vacuum environment removes all stain from the medullary canal via the drainage of the linea aspera

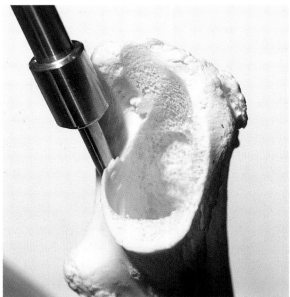

Fig. 133. The proximal cannula is placed in the fovea intertrochanterica and does not appear in the implant bed

instead of rasping and heparinization of the medullary canal, yielding a decrease in TEE-positive "events" from 94% in the control groups to 14% in the vacuum application groups. The step of controlled jet lavage together with 3%–5% H_2O_2 can probably further improve the results under such clinical evaluation (Pitto et al. 1998). The position of the proximal vacuum cannula was one of the essential factors in improving the prevention of embolic complication (Fig. 133). After the bone cement has been suctioned in by vacuum applied through the distal drill hole the proximal cannula must be held open. It lies in the intertrochanteric cancellous bone in alignment with the linea aspera and suctions out all the blood and bone marrow which gets pushed out during insertion of the stem. The proximal cannula remains free of bone cement because it is protected by the spongiosa of the proximal dorsal metaphysis. The cannulated screw is inserted in a 4.5-mm drill hole. Then the cannula is screwed into the spongiosa structure in such a way that its tip does not appear in the implant bed. A well-functioning suction through the proximal cannulated screw is considered to be the most important milestone to avoid thromboembolisms.

8.2
The Distal Drill Hole

The distal drill hole is the safest drainage of the medullary canal during THR (Breed 1974; Kallos et al. 1974; Ulrich et al. 1985; Ulrich1995). It can be considered an essential step of the procedure (Draenert 1989).

Tests with cannulated stems show that the drainage is insufficient, unreproducible and uncontrolled. Very often even blood cannot be suctioned off, but air; if so, foaming up of blood can occur in the medullary canal under vacuum conditions. The distal drill hole does not yield fatigue fractures if it is drilled 2 cm below the metal tip, if only one cortex is drilled and if cement filling of the hole is avoided by using a stopper acting as a filter at the level of the cannula.

In cadaver specimens it was found that firmly fixed components in the femur demonstrated a thin layer of fibrous tissue around the metal tip of the stem; 5 mm below, however, a thick fibrous tissue layer was pronounced; the physiological bending moment acting on the proximal femur shifts the moment to the level below the metal tip of the stem thus generating relative movements there which induce bone reabsorption and fibrous tissue formation; the layer's thickness corresponded directly to the relative motion between bone cement and bone (Draenert and Draenert 1992). Therefore 2 cm below the metal tip the drill hole is placed using a precise drill guide.

This was not observed in femurs with loose components.

All instruments are constructed to exclude endangering the patient. The special drill is held by the guide parallel while drilling; the tip of the trocar is steeply angled so that slipping does not occur.

The drill tip always reaches the center of the medullary canal if the jig is twisted 15° anteriorly from the exact lateral position. The penetration depth of the drill is limited so that drilling through the two cortices cannot occur.

With normal-thick cortices the self cutting cannula signals through its calibration when its tip appears in the medullary canal. The drill guide firmly fixed onto the bone the cannula is screwed in till the second bench mark reaches the guide; in this way the tube is protected from being torn out during manipulation of the leg.

Bone cement entering the drill hole is safely avoided due to the medullary cavity plug:

In order to blindly achieve these fast, reproducible and reliable results, a forged steel jig was constructed. This jig does not allow tangential drilling.

All instruments are constructed to exclude dangerous gambles.

A 1.5-mm Kirschner wire is inserted in the cannula during the setting of the medullary cavity plug (MCP): it signals the arrival of the MCP, now the cannula is twisted back to the first mark: the MCP can exceed 2.5 cm (no more). The cannula is now twisted up to the MCP and afterwards twisted back 1/4 revolution: now the MCP cannot distally dislocate; the cannula is not obstructed by the cement.

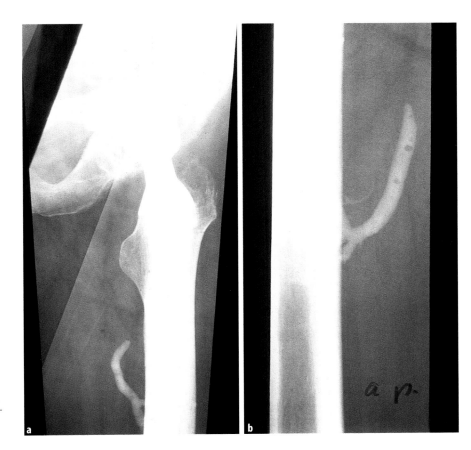

Fig. 134. Thick stems which are cemented press bone cement into the commitant veins of the nutrient artery

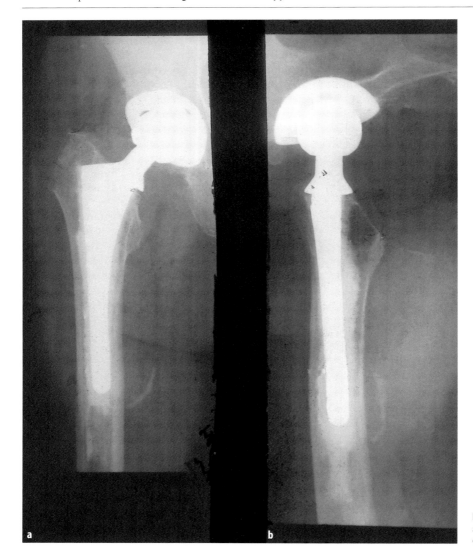

Fig. 135a,b. More cylindrical stems (cannulated) are more conflicting in this aspect

8.3
The Stem-Canal Volume Relationship

Dederich (1981) could demonstrate the cementing of vessels along the linea aspera in the lateral view of an X-ray. There is a stem-canal volume relationship which was found during the clinical thromboembolism study in patients in which a massive stem was implanted in a stove-pipe configurated canal. Regularly the commitant vein of the nutrient vessel was found to be filled even with a standard viscosity bone cement (Figs. 134, 135).

Cannulated stems (Schmidt 1996) which demonstrated a more cylindrical than conical configuration are considered to be more conflicting in that aspect.

CHAPTER 9
Consideration of the Prosthetic Design of the Femoral Stem

All long-term results of clinical follow-up studies (Wroblewski and Siney 1993; Older 1995) as well as the pathohistological studies (Draenert and Draenert 1992) show the superiority of delicate stems over massive constructions.

9.1
Stiffening Spongiosa of the Femur

The thorough study of the femur's reinforcing spongiosa in corroded and "defattened" sections by sequenced section analysis, and the digitilization of spongiosa compartments showed that the femur and its stiffened structures are torqued. The preservation of strong metaphyseal cancellous bone compartments and the integrity of the entire spongiosa in the diaphysis left a medullary cavity which represented a torqued space. This free space could be used for a prosthesis design without destroying the interior reinforcement of the femur.

The hourglasslike stiffening in the sagittal direction of a horizontal cross section stood out in the plateau of the center of rotation. A picture of a pendulum cogwheel (Fig. 136) corresponds to the gait analysis from "heel strike" to "toe off" phase.

The femoral neck section (Fig. 137) demonstrates strong bundles of trabeculae going round the Ward's zone; the strong spongiosa from the head formed the medial structure. The cortex fans out ventrally in a strong pattern toward the trochanteric massif. The strongest structures were found dorsally and these also fanned out to the trochanteric massif.

This U-shape of the stiffened area in the proximal femur must be preserved

In the plateau of the lesser trochanter (Fig. 138), the calcar femoris and the dorsal massif form a significant reinforced area. The ventral bundle forms an arc and leaves free space for the main mass of the prosthesis stem. The cross-section of the femur is almost rectangular.

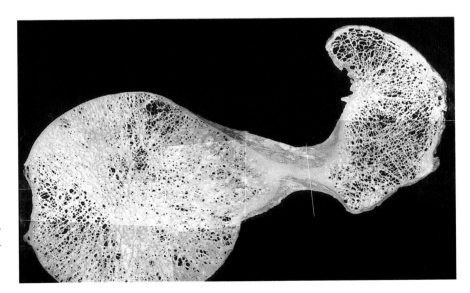

Fig. 136. The strong cancellous bone of the center of rotation is oriented in an externally rotated limb of the heelstrike phase in sagittal direction

Chapter 9 Consideration of the Prosthetic Design of the Femoral Stem

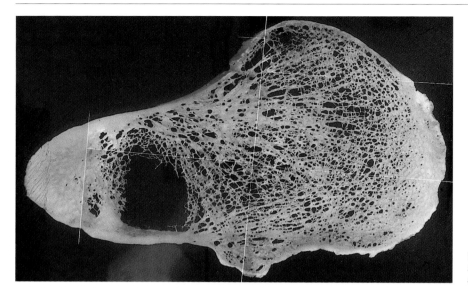

Fig. 137. The femoral neck section with strong anterior and posterior bundles

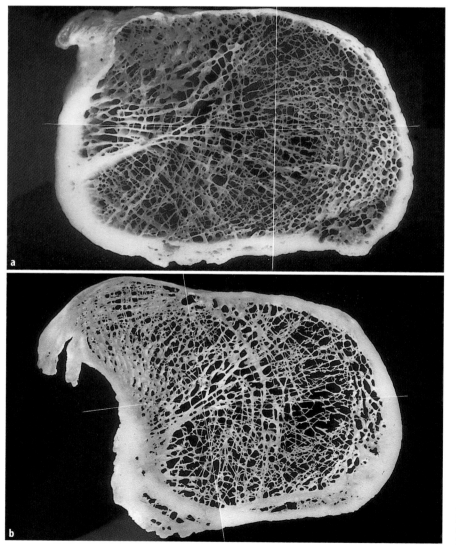

Fig. 138a–c. The calcar femoris and the dorsal compartment represent the strongest cancellous bone of the proximal metaphysis

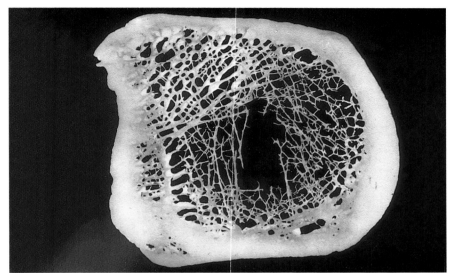

Fig. 138 c

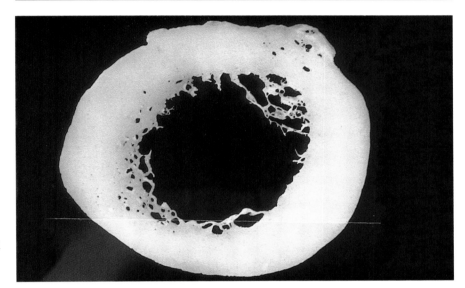

Fig. 139. The ellipsiform shape of the femoral cross-section twists from proximal to distal, from a frontal projection to a nearly sagittal orientation

9.2
Calcar Femoris

The calcar femoris (Bereiter et al. 1995; Merkel 1874) is the dorsal wall of the femoral neck and forms a very solid structure, and it represents the front compartment of the femoral cross-section of the proximal metaphysis. The preservation of the femoral neck and thus its dorsal wall, the calcar femoris, is of the utmost importance for rotational stability. A torqued femoral stem which passes through the femoral neck compartment shows two characteristics: first, it is curved anatomically following an anticurvature, and, second, it has a concave configuration on its dorsal side; thus it has kidney-like configurations in the complete cross-section. The stem can be twisted backward 15°–20° if the calcar femoris is removed. This rotation is prevented by its preservation. The femur's cross-section is oval, with the larger diameter in a frontal plane twisting to the sagittal plane distally (Figs. 139, 140).

Digitized cross-sections clearly show that the calcar femoris is also torqued. Stacking the cross-sections demonstrates that the prosthesis stem must follow the antecurvature of the femoral neck along its ventral wall if the dorsal wall is not to be destroyed. The structure of the calcar femoris allows adjustment of a kidneylike cross-section the main mass of which is projected laterally over the diaphyseal tube. Thus distribution of load is optimized into the proximal lumen (Figs. 140, 141).

The rectangular cross-section of the minor trochanter is followed by a cross-section which presents the long diameter in a frontal plane forming a frontal ellipsoid

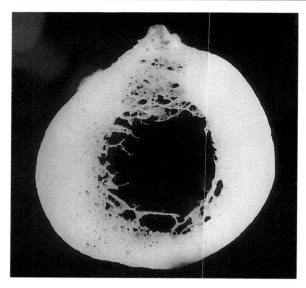

which twists over the length of the diaphysis into a sagittally oriented ellipsoid cross section. This leads to the specific interior reinforcement of the peripheral solid spongiosa. Therefore the spongiosa must be preserved.

The endosteal spongiosa of the diaphysis must be completely preserved. It forms the structure that allows the bone cement to interlock and it contributes essentially to the stiffening of the femoral bone. The three-dimensional reconstruction of the free space in the femoral cross-sections (Fig. 141) shows a torqued stem with a kidneylike cross-section proximally and a clearly ventral and lateral shift of its mass in relation to the construction axis (=femoral canal axis). Surprisingly, this constellation corresponds to perfect histological and clinical results from stems that were set in valgus position with lateralization of their mass.

Fig. 140. Sagitally oriented ellipsiform shape of the medullary cavity

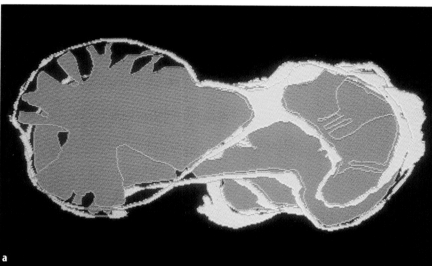

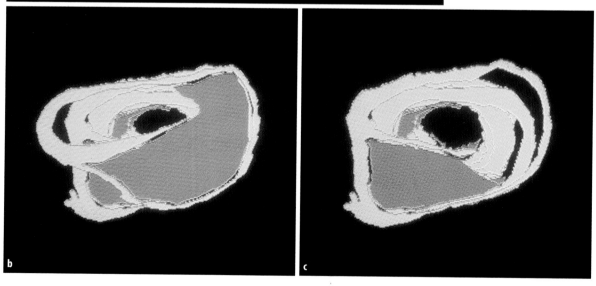

Fig. 141a–f. Torquing of the tube of the femur demonstrated by three-dimensional reconstruction of cross-sections

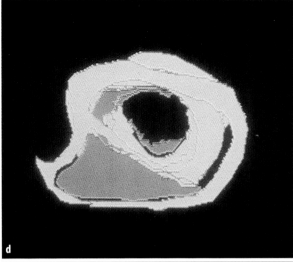

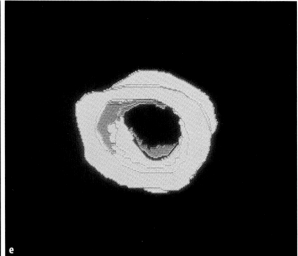

Fig. 141 d–f

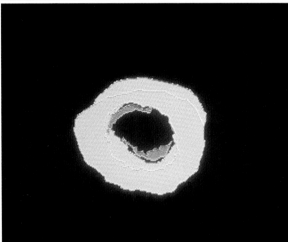

Fig. 142. Three-dimensional reconstruction of femoral cross-section demonstrating the antecurvature and the twist of the femoral tube

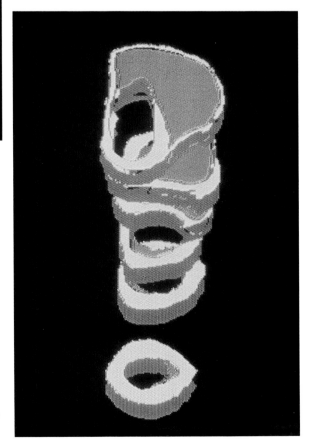

9.3
Stem Design

The prosthesis stem leaves the compartments of reinforcement of the femur intact and looks very similar to the Charnley type I stem. The stem's medial curvature originates from the study of the growth of the femoral neck and crosses the Shenton line. It ensures equal transmission of load. The offset of the prosthesis has been reduced to 40 mm in the standard stem in order to take into account the positive Charnley results by valgization (Older 1995) and histology. This leads to a medialization of the femur which clearly reduces the stress acting on the femoral anchorage. At the same time the standard prosthesis rebuilds the physiological height of the center of rotation (Fig. 142).

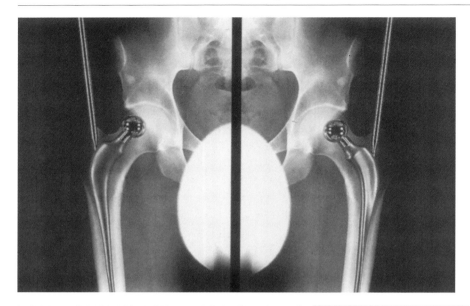

Fig. 143. Smart anatomical stem with 40-mm standard offset and straight implantation axis

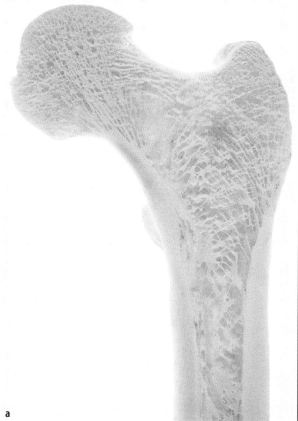

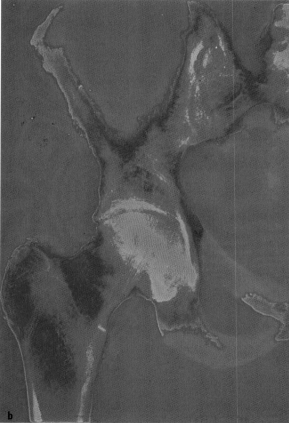

Fig. 144. a Sectioned and ground femur revealing the spongiosa honeycombs that line the medullary canual.

b "Alignment" can be demonstrated in a gray-contrast contour photograph of the hip joint with support structures expanding from the femur through the joint surface into the sacroiliac joint

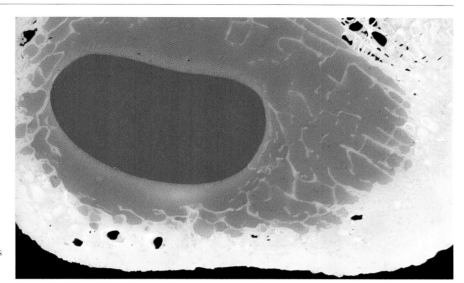

Fig. 145. Cross-section of an implanted anatomical CTS stem in the proximal metaphysis. The strong cancellous bone is preserved and stiffened by bone cement

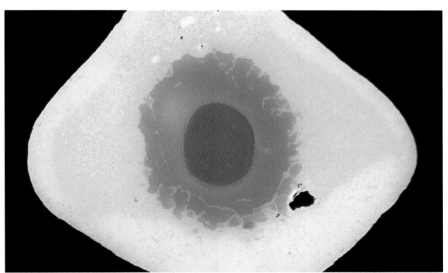

Fig. 146. The tip of the stem is centralized by preserving the cancellous bone deep in the diaphysis of the femur

Size 4 of these stems has an offset of 45 mm, which resulted from anatomic statistical data.

Viewed dorsally, the shaft shows certain characteristics that clearly differentiate it from the Charnley stem. It becomes apparent that the mass of the prosthesis was shifted proximally and ventrally. The distal stem remains delicate and adapts to any medullary canal thus leaving the bone structures unattached by rasps (Fig. 143).

The sectioned and ground femur shows stiffened structures in its frontal plane; the medial bundle runs to the joint surface. The strong spongiosa honeycombs that line the medullary canal are clearly visible (Fig. 144a).

What is described with the term "alignment," can be demonstrated in the gray-contrast contour photograph of the hip joint; supporting structures expand from the femur through the joint surface into the sacroiliac joint (Fig. 144 b).

The stem, which can be implanted without rasping the strong cancellous bone, is self-centralized by the preserved bony structure proximally (Fig. 145) and distally as well (Fig. 146).

9.4
Preoperative Planning

The preoperative planning must take into account the anatomy of the femur and the anatomy of the acetabulum. When determining the rotation center in the femur one must consider that the femoral head is already free of cartilage and is in an advanced state of deformation as seen in the X-ray. From the study by Noble et al. (1988) and from our own measurements it can be concluded that no correlation can be established between the anatomy of the medullary canal and the offset (lever arm to the center of rotation), or between the antetorsion and the weight bearing joint surface. Concerning the cemented component, one must ensure that the distal femur is not rasped at all and that the femoral neck compartment is preserved with the help of the SDI technique. Histomorphological studies show that bony contact with the prosthesis can be achieved in a dorsal, medial, or anteromedial U-shape and that large surfaces must be provided.

9.4.1
Plane of the Metaphyseal "V"

An interesting correlation was found in the series that we conducted, one between a plane laid down onto the metaphysis and the position of the center of rotation (elevation of about 25 mm; 1.15:1). The plane of the open metaphysis is defined by the endpoint of the diaphyseal-metaphyseal funnel; laterally by the innominate tubercle, and the inner Shenton line medially. A ray departing from the innominate tubercle set tangentially to the inner Shenton line defines in the frontal X-ray in the metaphyseal plane two-dimensionally. The construction axis of the prosthesis (=canal axis of the femur) is the guideline for implantation. It crosses the metaphyseal plane and defines the implant and the implantation. The formation of the Shenton line can be traced through animal experiments studying the formation of the femoral neck by polychromatic fluorescence labeling (Draenert and Draenert 1995). In an axial view of an X-ray the posterior wall of the neck of the calcar femoris is aligned to the dorsal wall of the canal line. Thus prosthesis stems which are so delicate that rasping of the medullary canal is avoided do not need a S-shape configuration in order to centralize themselves in the medullary canal. This brings important advantages in setting and removing prosthesis stems. In studies of cadaver femora a good correlation was established between the metaphyseal plane and the position of the center of rotation (mean elevation 25 mm).

The femoral canal axis and the metaphyseal plane are marked. If the angle is smaller than 4° opposing the femoral canal axis, a coxa vara is present. If the angle is greater than 7° a coxa valga is diagnosed (Fig. 147).

The 1.15:1 line graph is superimposed taking care that stems and canal axis are coincident and the medial edge lies on the metaphyseal plane (MP). According to the uncorrected metaphyseal plane a coxa vara or valga position remains unchanged, e.g., coxa vara in Fig. 148.

The stem design considers a MP of 7°. If this angle is applied, the center of rotation is reconstructed; the resultant force "R" is nicely aligned in most cases to the sacroiliac joint (Fig. 149).

The complete construction before surgery demonstrates a medialization due to the shortening of the offset, showing, however, reestablishment of normal leg length (Fig. 150).

9.4.2
Offset and Alignment

In his book, Charnley expressed doubt about his chosen offset of 45 mm. He did not have the opportunity, as did Older (1995), to conduct 20- to 25-year follow-ups of his surgeries and to evaluate the results. All cases demonstrated by Older had a 40- to 42-mm offset. Charnley arrived at this empirically by implanting his prosthesis in valgus position. It was shown histologically that a Müller banana stem implanted in valgus position had a very good long lasting result (Draenert and Draenert 1992).

Careful preoperative planning shows that the femoral neck is set into the small basin with a CCD angle of 120°. This explains the inevitable complications of the cup anchorage with displacement into the small basin in Charnley's patients (Charnley 1979). "Alignment" refers to the orientation of the resultant force (femoral neck of the prosthesis) directed toward the sacroiliac joint. With an offset of 40 mm this alignment can be regularly achieved (femoral neck angle 135°). The offset is adapted to the specific anatomy (Fig. 151).

Furthermore, comparative measurements of cadaver femora demonstrated that the isthmus of the femur (the narrowest point in the diaphyseal tube) varies. The length of the stem must not go beyond the isthmus, for the isthmus represents the curvature's strongest point. There was no significant correlation between the isthmus of the prosthesis and other measurements of the femoral medullary canal in the series by Noble et al. (1988) nor in our statistics. Sections of the spongiosa honeycomb rows along the inner wall of the medullary canal in the 17–21 cm area (starting from the middle of the intertrochanteric line) were 3, sometimes 4, and rarely 2 mm thick. Using a 3-mm cement layer, a size 1 stem could be implanted in 60% of the cases, and a size 2 stem in another 20%. Otherwise the layer thickness of the bone cement in A-P projection would have exceeded 3 mm. The remaining 20% used sizes 3, 4, and in narrower lavities type 0 or even –1.

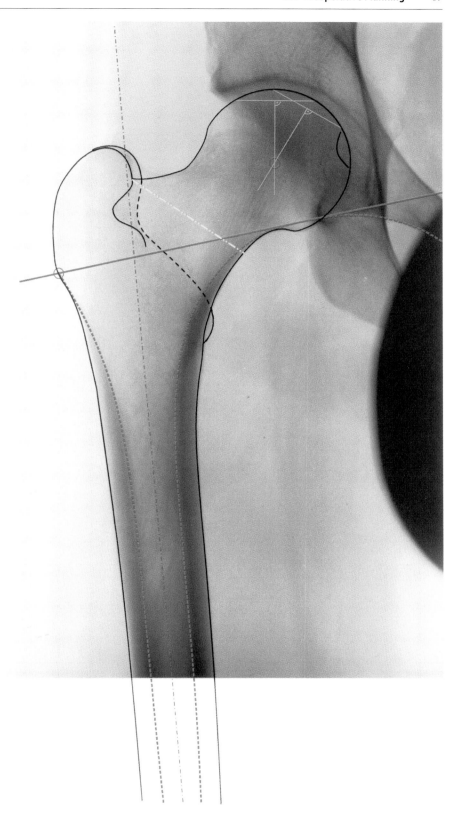

Fig. 147. Drawing of a preoperative planning on an X-ray, demonstrating the femoral canal axis and the metaphyseal plane

88 Chapter 9 **Consideration of the Prosthetic Design of the Femoral Stem**

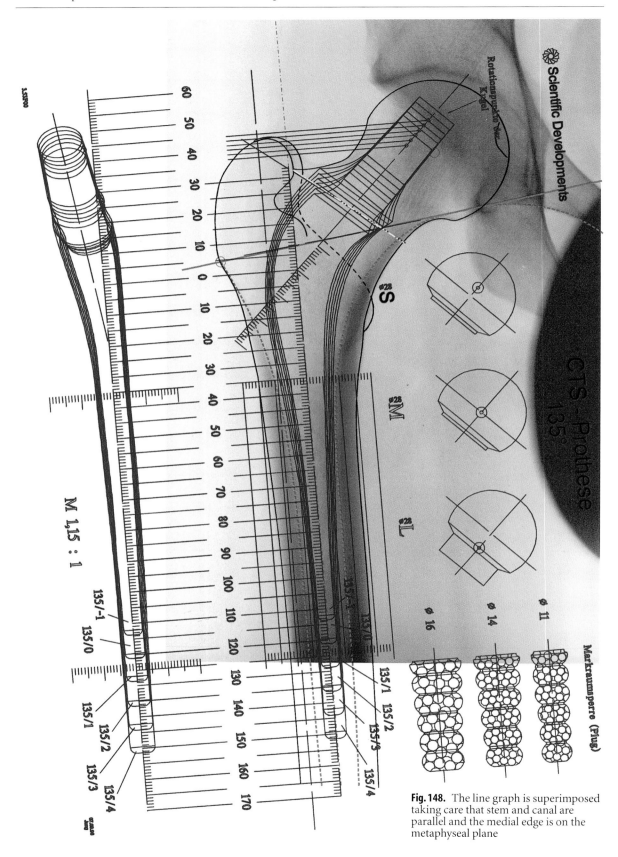

Fig. 148. The line graph is superimposed taking care that stem and canal are parallel and the medial edge is on the metaphyseal plane

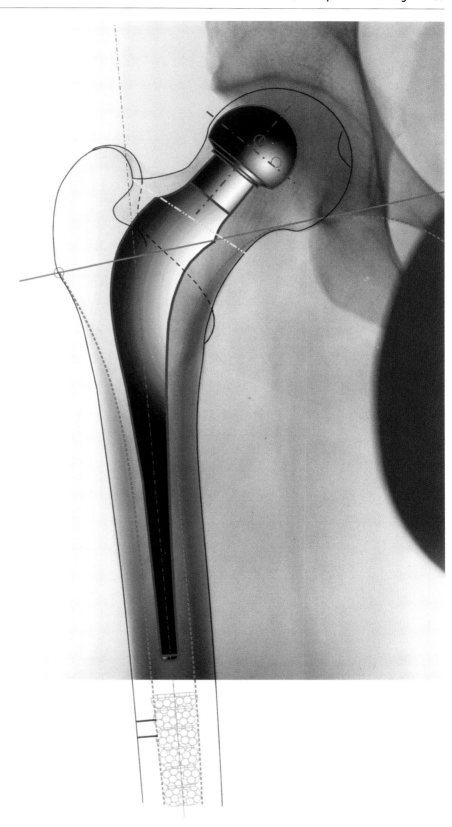

Fig. 149. Reconstruction of the center of rotation

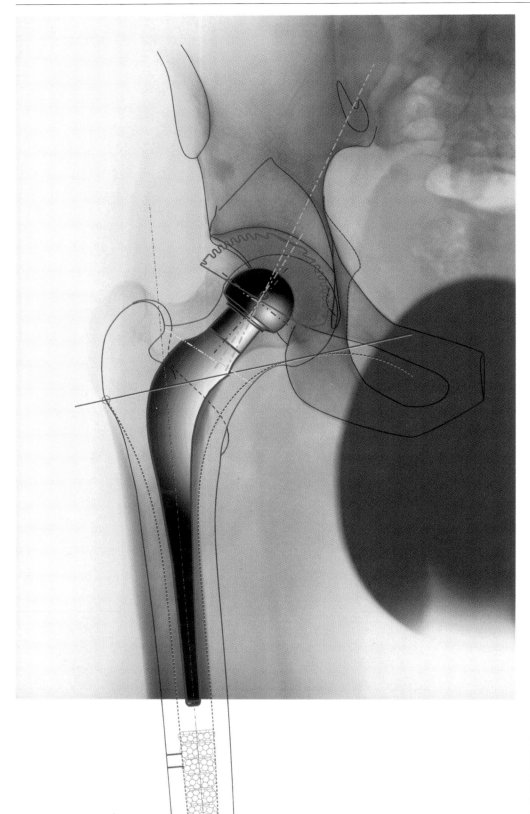

Fig. 150. Complete construction with cup and repositioning reveals the medialization due to the short offset

9.4 Preoperative Planning 91

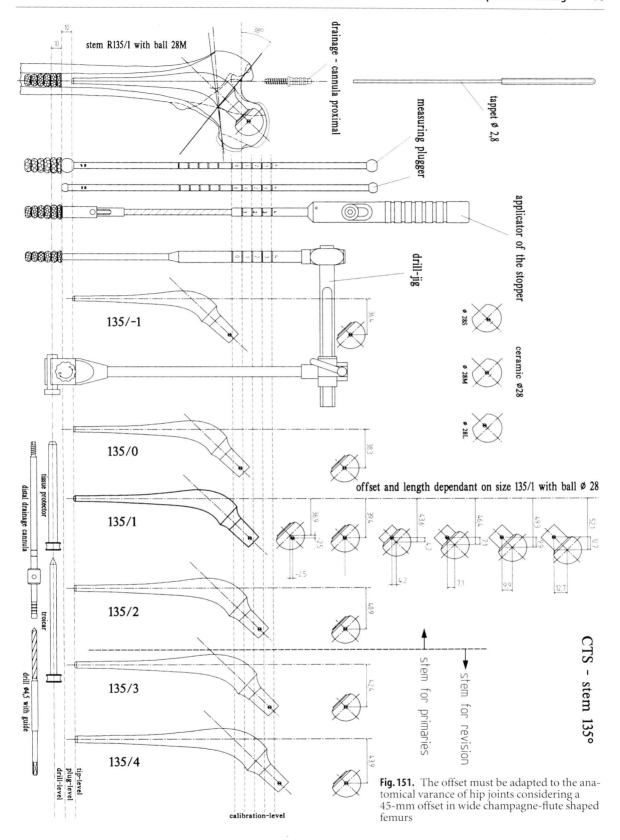

Fig. 151. The offset must be adapted to the anatomical varance of hip joints considering a 45-mm offset in wide champagne-flute shaped femurs

9.5
Centralizing Anatomical Design

Replicas of the stems were implanted into 20 femora, after preoperative planning, using the previously described technique. In all cases it was found that over the entire length of the prosthesis it was centered. The peripheral spongiosa was preserved and the calcar femoris was undamaged. Furthermore, the cement border was formed artefact-free along the entire length of the prosthesis.

The kidneylike cross-section of the stem adapted nicely to the ventral wall of the femur and preserves the spongiosa and the femoral neck (Fig. 145).

One of the most interesting observations during clinical validation was the self-centering of the shaft in the preserved spongiosa structures. The tip of the prosthesis is guided by the preserved spongiosa and always settles centrally. The interlocking cement is clearly seen (Fig. 146).

The anatomy of the stem takes into account the femoral neck compartment and shows a ventral curvature. The mass of the stem is shifted towards the femoral tube thus transferring the load more equally into the femur.

The medial curvature of the prosthesis crosses the Shenton line directly below the osteotomy. This does not allow the stem's subsiding but does ensure an even load transmission to the proximal femur. The curvature originates from studies on the growth and formation of the femoral neck in animals (Draenert and Draenert 1995). The labels indicate new bone formation along the endosteal surface of the medullary canal. Forming the neck they cross the spongiosa framework of the proximal metaphysis. The extension of the femoral neck occurs while at the same time the next plateau of the growth plate is formed. According to the Shenton's curve load from the hip joint is equally transmitted into the bone structure.

CHAPTER 10
Instrumentation

Quick and purposeful use of instruments necessitates the use of an instrumentation table with a working area for the surgeon and a working area for the nurse equipped with a vacuum pump for both (Fig. 152). The instruments were placed in a central position so they were easily accessible to both (Fig. 153).

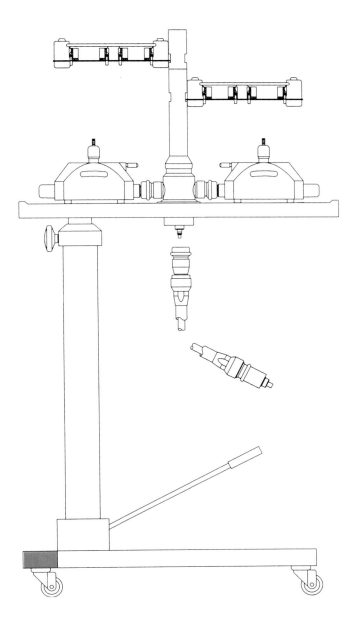

Fig. 152. Modular instrumentation table prepared for the vacuum technique

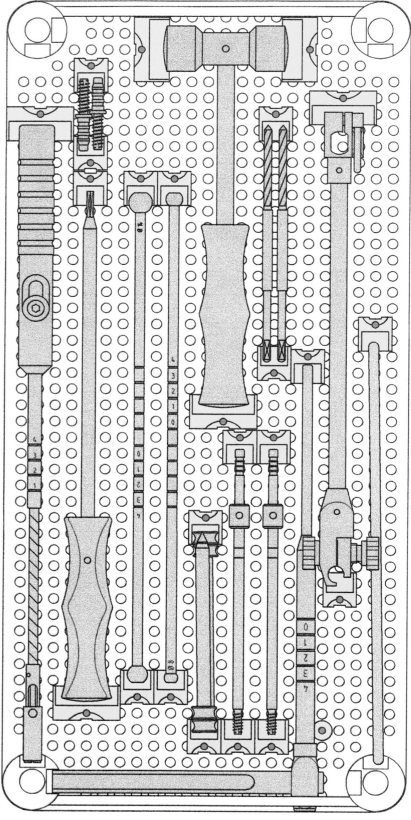

Fig. 153 a,b. All instruments are prepared in the steri tray ready for use on the evening before the operation

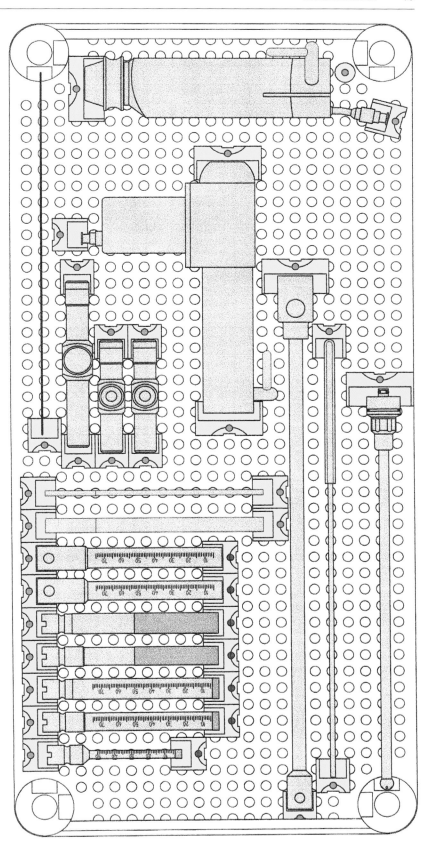

Fig. 153 b

CHAPTER 11
Conclusions: The Success of Cemented Components

The success of Charnley type I prostheses in place for more than 15 years and up to 26 years has been reported by many study groups (Table 8).

Table 8. Long-term success of Charnley type I prostheses

Reference	Duration (years)
Clarac (1995)	20
Kavanagh et al. (1994)	20
Kavanagh et al. (1989)	15
Lazcano et al. (1995)	20–25
Lewalle et al. (1995)	20
Madey et al. (1997)	20
Neumann et al. (1994)	15–20
Older (1995)	25
Schulte et al. (1993)	20
Wroblewski (1986)	15–21
Wroblewski et al. (1992)	19–25

Clinical studies are revealing a relationship between improved cementing techniques and a decrease in revision rates that is impressive as it is published by the group in Rochester. Beckenbaugh and Ilstrup (1978) reported a four-to-seven year follow-up with Charnley's low-friction (CLF) arthroplasties and determined a loosening rate of 24%, according to X-ray findings. Russotti et al. (1988) published a follow-up of CLF arthroplasties 5–7 years after the operation in which the so-called second-generation cementing technique was applied. In these operations a stopper was introduced and the medullary cavity was filled with a low viscosity bone cement in a retrograde manner after the canal was cleaned with a pulsatile lavage. Russotti et al. findings using the same examination procedure and scores as Beckenbaugh and Ilstrup (1978) were 1.2% definitive, 0.4% potential and 0.8% possible loosenings, yielding an overall loosening rate of 2.4%. The authors concluded that improved cementing techniques were seven to ten times more effective as a result of interlocking.

An evaluation conducted by the Swedish National Health Register emphasizes the success of cemented in comparison to noncemented designs (Herberts et al. 1989; Malchau et al. 1993; Malchau and Herberts 1996). The cement free PCA stem reveals a steep increase in revisions, and the smart cemented Charnley I crosses the stronger and heavier Lubinus after the 10th year. The conclusion that can be drawn is: only smart stems reached 15–25 years results.

Why are cemented femoral components more successful than cement-free procedures?

With cement-free components, metal-to-bone load transfer produces deformation, excessive deformation generates relative movement, and relative movement yields bone reabsorption and developing of tight fibrous tissue (Draenert and Draenert 1992). We can conclude the following:

- Cancellous bone cannot carry the load.
- Cancellous bone must be removed!
- "The myth of press-fit" of Noble et al. (1988) showed clearly that in all cement-free procedures the load is transferred in a very restricted area thus producing a stress concentration.
- One circumscribed part of bone hypertrophies, and the rest becomes severely osteoporotic.
- Only a limited number of femurs providing an adequate anatomy can be operated without bone cement.

With cemented components, on the other hand, we observe that:

- Stiffened cancellous bone resists deformation.
- They distribute load equally.
- They thus avoid bone atrophy.
- They avoid stress concentration.
- They guarantee a tolerance in the procedure, and with respect to the surgeon and the individual bone.
- The success of cemented components depends on the cementing technique.

11.1
First-Generation Cementing Techniques

Charnley described the conventional cementing technique, including curettage (6 in. in length), mixing bone cement to produce a stiff dough. A sausage-shaped form was modeled from the dough, the cavity was suctioned, and the bone cement impacted using a finger packing technique.

The main steps of the second-generation cementing technique were the introduction of a stopper and the jet lavage (Amstutz et al. 1976; Miller and Serot 1978; Oh et al. 1978). Miller and Serot (1978) showed that cleaning was important. The basic study that underscored the importance of a lavage procedure was conducted by the group in Toronto (Sherman et al. 1983). Based on their experiments it was concluded that using a stopper, performing a lavage, and injecting a low viscosity hand-mixed bone cement in a retrograde manner must be understood as second-generation cementing technique (Ballard et al. 1994).

It was also understood that interlocking of bone cement was the important result for these improvements (Markolf and Amstutz 1976a,b) and bleeding was the limiting factor (Benjamin et al. 1987; Halawa et al. 1978). It has never been confirmed that a low viscosity bone cement has actually been helpful in improving the anchorage of a component. A low viscosity bone cement has a low penetration capacity, high miscibility, a steep polymerization curve related to a low tolerance of the procedure (Draenert and Draenert 1988). Based on the studies in which penetration was measured as pressure dependent (Halawa et al. 1978; Maloney et al. 1996), a completely new technique had been introduced to increase longevity of the anchorage (Benjamin et al. 1987; Draenert and Draenert 1988; Halawa et al. 1978; Harris 1980; Krause et al. 1982; Markolf and Amstutz 1976b; Weinstein et al. 1976). It was not clearly defined whether the "high-pressurize technique" is considered a third-generation cementing technique, or whether it was to a certain degree already included in the second-generation cementing technique (Ballard et al. 1994). A more precise definition of these three categories was offered by the Swedish study (Malchau et al. 1993):

- The old technique means no plug, no seal, no compression, hand mixing of bone cement, no cleaning of the medullary canal
- Early techniques comprise plug, hand mixing, brush and a retrograde filling as recommended by Harris and McGann (1986).
- Modern techniques use vacuum mixing, brush and pulsatile lavage (Malchau and Herberts 1996), sealing, and pressurizing of bone cement, retrograde filling. This technique may be considered the third-generation cementing technique.

It was clearly shown that "modern" ("third-generation") cementing techniques had the best results at a stage between the sixth and seventh years in the Swedish study (Malchau and Herberts 1996). The Swedish National Hip Arthroplasty Register (SNHAR; Malchau and Herberts 1996) is impressive. There is, however, a need for a more practicable procedure for predicting the final outcome and prognosis of one step of improvement at an earlier stage. Migration and subsidence were considered in order to predict the loosening of a component and approaches were discussed to measure the two phenomena accurately. The EBRA method and radio-stereogrammetry, although more complicated, but more precise with a higher resolution, were introduced (Balderson et al. 1979; Bylander et al. 1981; Kärrholm et al. 1982, 1994; Lindstrand and Selvik 1976; Mjöber et al. 1984; Mogensen et al. 1982; Olsson et al. 1976; Russe 1988; Ryd et al. 1983; Ryd 1986; Selvik 1974; Selvik et al. 1985; Tjörnstrand et al. 1981). Progressive migration is considered a sign of loosening (Ryd 1986). The radio-stereogrammetry, however, cannot answer the question of whether bone is equally loaded via a large surface and why bone disappears.

11.2
Success of the Cemented Component Is Due to Stiffened Bone Structures

The last and best and most precise answer to the question of how bone responds to an implant is given by a three-dimensional histological assay of the implant as a whole or even whole articulation (Draenert and Draenert 1992).

First, "fibrocartilage" (Charnley 1970a) was reported as normal tissue in the interface between bone cement and bone. The bone-to-cement contact was then systematically analyzed, and fibrous-tissue free contacts were presented (Draenert et al. 1976; Draenert and Rudigier 1978; Malcolm 1990). Even in the transmission electron microscope, fibrous-tissue-free contacts were published (Linder and Hansson 1983). The success of cemented components was in all cases due to preserved bone structures stiffened by bone cement and protected from stress shielding (Draenert and Draenert 1992; Jasty et al. 1990; Maloney et al. 1996).

11.3
Cancellous Bone Stiffened by Bone Cement Can Survive

It has been reported that bony trabeculae embedded in bone cement atrophy and are replaced by fibrous tissue (Bloebaum et al. 1984; Goodman et al. 1985; Hoy et al. 1984; Shao et al. 1993). The histology presented by Draenert and Draenert 1992, however, did not confirm these studies. In all four studies, the experimental model chosen was an implantation of bone cement into the metaphysis. It is, however, a well-known fact that a load can be transmitted from a joint surface by bypassing a metaphyseal implant. As a result, bony atrophy and replacement of the embedded trabeculae by fibrous tissue due to stress protection occurs (Goodman et al. 1985).

Epiphyseal cancellous bone embedded in bone cement does not atrophy and reveals two very interesting features: there is no heat necrosis and, due to shrinkage of bone cement, a very fast revascularization was observed along the interface (Draenert and Draenert 1992). A single honeycomb has a diameter of 500–1000 µm and a PMMA ball with that diameter does not generate heat. Due to shrinkage of the cold polymerizing material, a gap has been formed in a three-dimensional pattern in which vessels can grow rapidly, forming a capillary network. After 1 year a good symbiosis between bone and bone cement has been observed. Remodeling and even reabsorption can be detected along the interface at an early stage because a fast revascularization was observed in the gap formed by the shrinkage (Draenert and Draenert 1992).

11.4
Preservation of Cancellous Bone

Charnley's relationship (Charnley 1953) to cancellous bone was influenced by an observation of the gap healing of an arthrodesis which revealed a shift of the weight-bearing axis. Charnley wrote, "I now believe that cancellous bone even with an intact blood supply has in fact a very restricted form of osteogenetic activity." For cementation of femoral components, he requested, "The curettage is pursued until all cancellous bone has been removed from the medullary canal and especially from the medial, anterior and posterior walls." His conclusions can be summarized simply as "cancellous bone cannot carry the load." In all operating theaters around the world, rasping the canal of the femur is the method of choice for preparing it for the stem. Many surgeons are using the largest rasp that would fit readily (Harris and McGann 1986). Müller (1975) and Charnley (1979) used a straight rasp for an S-shaped femoral canal, thus preserving distinct areas of cancellous bone. Interlocking of bone cement in these cancellous bone honeycombs explains the good results which were shown histologically (Draenert and Draenert 1992). The atraumatic preparation of bone necessitates a wet-grinding procedure (Draenert 1988), using the diamond technique for opening and preparation of the medullary canal. In this way both the framework and the vasculature of the cancellous bone of the metaphysis are preserved (Breusch et al. 1998).

The distal tube of the femur should not be touched at all. A smart stem is therefore requested. Leaving cancellous bone of the diaphysis unattached guarantees a centralization of the stem as well as a deep interlocking of bone cement along the diaphyseal cortex (Breusch et al. 1998).

References

Alho A, Hoiseth A, Husby T (1988) Bone density and bone strength – an ex vivo study on cadaver femora. Rev Chir Orthop 74:333–334

Amstutz HC, Markolf KL, McNeise GM, Gruen TA (1976) Loosening of total hip components: cause and prevention. The Hip Society. Proceedings of the fourth open scientific meeting. Mosby, St Louis, pp 102–116

Anderson LD, Hamsa WR, Waring FL (1964) Femoral-head prostheses. J Bone Joint Surg Am 46:1049–1065

Aufranc OE (1957) Constructive hip surgery with the Vitallium mold. J Bone Joint Surg Am 39:237–248

Balderson H, Egund N, Hannson LI, Selvik G (1979) Instability and wear of total hip prosthesis determined with roentgen stereophotgrammetry. Arch Orthop Traumat Surg 95:257–263

Ballard WT, Callaghan JJ, Sullivan PM, Johnston RC (1994) The results of improved cementing techniques for total hip arthroplasty in patients less than fifty years old. J Bone Joint Surg Am 76:959–964

Barton JR (1827) On the treatment of ankylosis by the formation of artificial joints. North Am Med Surg J 3:279

Bauer R, Kerschbaumer F, Poisel S (1986) Operative Zugangswege in Orthopädie und Traumatologie. Thieme, Stuttgart

Beckenbaugh RD, Ilstrup DM (1978) Total hip arthroplasty. A review of three hundred and thirty-three cases with long follow-up. J Bone Joint Surg Am 60:306–313

Beisaw NE, Comerota AJ, Groth HE, Merli GJ, Weitz HH, Zimmermann RC, Diserio FJ, Sasahara AA (1988) Dihydroergotamin/Heparin in the prevention of deep vein thrombosis after total hip replacement. J Bone Joint Surg Am 70:2–10

Bell RS, Schatzker J, Fornasier VL, Goodman SB (1985) A study of implant failure in the Wagner resurfacing arthroplasty. J Bone Joint Surg Am 67:1165

Benjamin JB, Gie GA, Lee AJC, Ling RSM (1987) Cementing technique and the effect of bleeding. J Bone Joint Surg Br 69:620–624

Bereiter H, Huggler AH, Gautier E (1995) Calcar femorale: eine bedeutende Struktur des Schenkelhalses. In: Draenert K (ed) Histo-Morphologie des Bewegungsapparates 4. Art and Science, Munich

Blacker GJ, Charnley J (1978) Changes in the upper femur after low friction arthroplasty. Clin Orthop 137:15–23

Bloebaum RD, Gruen TA, Sarmiento A (1984) Interface and bone response to increased penetration of bone cement. Trans Biomaterials 84:82

Bogner C, Landauer B (1991) Anaesthesiologische Aspekte bei Hüftprothesenoperationen. Presented at the 45th Praktischen Seminar in der Orthopädie und Chirurgie des Bewegungsapparates, 21 May 1991, Munich

Borris LC, Christiansen HM, Lassen MR, Olsen AD, Schött P (1989) Comparison of real-time b-mode ultrasonography and bilateral ascending phlebography for detection of postoperative deep vein thrombosis following elective hip surgery. Thrombosis Haemost 61:363–365

Brady LP, McCutchen JW (1986) A ten-year follow-up study of 170 Charnley total hip arthroplasties. Clin Orthop 211:51–54

Breed AL (1974) Experimental production of vascular hypotension and bone marrow and fat embolism with methylmethacrylate cement. Traumatic hypertension of bone. Clin Orthop 102:227–244

Breusch S (1993) Remodelingcharakteristik des knöchernen Lagers in Abhängigkeit von der Implantatoberfläche. Thesis, University of Munich

Breusch SJ, Draenert K, Draenert Y, Boerner M, Pitto RP (1998) Die anatomische Basis des zementierten Femurstieles. Z Orthop (in print)

Brighton CT, Strafford B, Gross SB (1991) The proliferative and synthetic response of isolated calvarial bone cells of rats to cyclic biaxial mechanical strain. J Bone Joint Surg Am 73:320–331

Brown AM (1947) Sculptured synthetic prostheses as implants in plastic surgery. Arch Otolaryng 45:339

Buchholz T (1992) Histomorphologische Untersuchungen zum Oberflächenersatz des Hüftgelenkes. Thesis, University of Munich

Burgess DM (1970) Cardiac arrest and bone cement. BMJ 3:588

Bylander B, Selvik G, Hansson LI, Aronsson S (1981) A roentgen stereophotogrammetric analysis of growth arrest by stapling. J Pediatr Orthop 1:81–90

Carter SR, Pynsent PB, McMinn DWJ (1990) Greater than ten year survivorship of Charnley low friction arthroplasty. J Bone Joint Surg Br 73:71

Charnley J (1953) Compression arthrodesis. Including central dislocation as a principle in hip surgery. Livingstone, Edinburgh

Charnley J (1960) Anchorage of the femoral head prosthesis to the shaft of the femur. J Bone Joint Surg Br 42:28–30

Charnley J (1961a) Arthroplasty of the hip. Lancet 1:1129–1132

Charnley J (1961b) The closed treatment of common fractures. Livingstone, Edinburgh

Charnley J (1964) The bonding of prostheses to bone by cement. J Bone Joint Surg Br 46:518

Charnley J (1970a) The reaction of bone to self-curing acrylic cement. J Bone Joint Surg Br 52:340

Charnley J (1970b) Acrylic cement in orthopaedic surgery. Livingstone, Edinburgh

Charnley J (1970c) Total hip replacement. Clin Orthop 72:1

Charnley J (1979) Low friction arthroplasty of the hip: theory and practice. Springer, Berlin Heidelberg New York

Charnley J, Crawford WJ (1968) Histology of bone in contact with self-curing cement. J Bone Joint Surg Br 50:228

Charnley J, Follacci FM, Hammond BT (1968) The long term reaction of bone to self-curing acrylic cement. J Bone Joint Surg Br 52:340

Chen PC, Pinto JG, Mead EH, D'Lima DD, Colwell CW (1997) Fatigue model to characterize cement-metal interface in dynamic shear. Clin Orthop 350:229–236

Ciarelli MJ, Goldstein SA, Dickie D, Ku JL, Kapper M, Stanley J, Flynn MJ, Matthews LS (1986) Experimental determination of the orthogonal mechanical properties, density and distribution of human trabecular bone from the major metaphyseal regions utilizing material testing and computed tomography. Orthop Trans 10:238

Claes L, Faiss S, Gerngross H, Wilke HJ (1990) Morphological changes in femoral heads following double-cup arthroplasty. In: Heimke G, Soltesz U, Lee AJC (eds) Clinical implant materials; advances in biomaterials, vol 9. Elsevier, Amsterdam, pp 403–408

Clarac JP (1995) Total hip implantation according to Charnley, 20 years ago. Charnley total hip arthroplasty. In: ACORA Group (ed) Charnley total hip arthroplasty. Transit Communications, Lyon

Clarius M (1996) Intraoperativer Embolienachweis mittels zweidimensionaler transösophagealer Echokardiographie beim künstlichen Hüftgelenkersatz. Thesis, University of Munich

Clarke MT, Green JS, Harper WM, Gregg PJ (1997) Screening for deep-venous thrombosis after hip and knee replacement without prophylaxis. J Bone Joint Surg Br 79:787–791

Cohen CA, Smith TC (1971) The intraoperative hazard of acrylic bone cement: report of a case. Anesthesiology 35:547–549

Convery FR, Gunn DR, Hughes JD, Martin WE (1975) The relative safety of polymethylmethacrylate. J Bone Joint Surg Am 57:57–64

Cook SD, Thomas KA, Haddad RJ Jr (1991) Histologic analysis of retrieved porous-coated human total joint components. Orthop 2:167–171

Currey JD (1984) Effects of differences in mineralization on the mechanical properties of bone. Philos Trans R Soc Lond 304:509–518

Dall DM (1975) Charnley hip replacements – early results. J Bone Joint Surg Br 57:259

Dall DM, Grobbelaar CJ, Learmonth ID, Dall G (1986) Charnley low-friction arthroplasty of the hip. Clin Orthop 211:85–90

Dandy DJ (1971) Fat embolism following prosthetic replacement of the femoral head. Injury 3:85–88

Daniel WW, Coventry MB, Miller WE (1972) Pulmonary complications after total hip arthroplasty with Charnley prosthesis as revealed by chest roentgenograms. J Bone Joint Surg Am 54: 282–283

Davis FM, Laurensen VG, Gillespie WJ, Wells JE, Foate J, Newman E (1988) Deep vein thrombosis after total hip replacement. J Bone Joint Surg Br 71:181–185

DeAngelis J, Kenneth J (1973) Cardiac arrest following acrylic-cement implants. Anaesth Analg 52:298–302

Delling G, Reichelt A, Engelbrecht E (1984) Knochen- und Grenzschichtveränderungen nach Implantation von Double-Cup Arthroplastiken. Z Orthop 122:770–776

Demarest VA, Lautenschlager EP, Wixon RL (1983) Vacuum mixing of acrylic bone cement. Presented at the 9th Annual Meeting of the Society for Biomaterials, Birmingham, Alabama, p 37

Dorr LD, Sakimura I, Mohler JG (1979) Pulmonary emboli following total hip arthroplasty: incidence study. J Bone Joint Surg Am 61:1083–1087

Draenert K (1981) Histomorphology of the bone-to-cement interface: remodeling of the cortex and revascularization of the medullary canal in animal experiments. The John Charnley Award Paper Chapter 7:71–109

Draenert K (1983) Forschung und Fortbildung in der Chirurgie des Bewegungsapparates 1. Zur Technik der Zementverankerung. Art and Science Munich

Draenert K (1986) Histomorphological observations on experiments to improve the bone-to-cement contact. Nicholas Andry – Award Paper Presented at the 38th Annual Meeting of the Association of Bone and Joint Surgeons, Vancouver, 27–31 March 1986

Draenert K (1989) Modern cementing techniques. An experimental study of vacuum insertion of bone cement. Acta Orthop Belg 55: 273–293

Draenert K (1988) Zur Praxis der Zementverankerung. In: Draenert K (ed) Forschung und Fortbildung in der Chirurgie des Bewegungsapparates 2. Art and Science, Munich

Draenert K (1990) Morphology of implant-bone interface in cemented and non-cemented endoprostheses. In: Older J (ed) Implant bone interface. Springer, Berlin Heidelberg New York, pp 27–34

Draenert K, Draenert Y (1984) Der Knochen als hydraulisches System. In: Frei O (ed) Subjektive Standorte in Baukunst und Naturwissenschaft IL 36. Krämer, Stuttgart, pp 108–109

Draenert K, Draenert Y (1987) Ein neues Verfahren für die Knochenbiopsie und die Knorpel-Knochen-Transplantation. Sandorama 2:31–38

Draenert K, Draenert Y (1992) Die Adaptation des Knochens an die Deformation durch Implantate. Strain adaptive bone remodelling. Art and Science, Munich

Draenert K, Draenert Y (1995) Die Bedeutung der Blutgefässe auf beiden Seiten der Wachstumsfuge. Orthopäde 24:394–401

Draenert K, Draenert Y (1996) Validierung der Zementiertechnik. Munich, Zentrum für Orthopädische Wissenschaften

Draenert K, Rudigier J (1978) Histomorphologie des Knochen-Zement-Kontaktes. Eine tierexperimentelle Phänomenologie der knöchernen Umbauvorgänge. Chirurg 49:276–285

Draenert K, Rudigier J, Willenegger H (1976) Tierexperimentelle Studie zur Histomorphologie des Knochen-Zement-Kontaktes. Helv Chir Acta 43:769–773

Draenert K, Ulrich C (1989) Die Thromboemboliekomplikation der Hüftgelenks-Endoprothesen Operation. Theodor Nägeli Preis

Drinker H, Panjabi M, Goel V (1981) Acute cardiopulmonary toxicity of methylmethacrylate pressurization in the dog femur. Ortho Trans 5:275–276

Eftekhar NS (1971) Charnley low friction torque arthroplasty. A study of long-term results. Clin Orthop 81:93

Eftekhar NS, Tzitzikalakis GI (1986) Failures and reoperations following low-friction arthroplasty of the hip. A five to fifteen-year follow-up study. Clin Orthop 211:65–78

Eftekhar NS (1987) Long-term results of cemented total hip arthroplasty. Clin Orthop 225:207–217

Egbert R, Hundelshausen B von, Gradinger R, Hipp E, Kolb E (1989) Herzstillstand bei Implantation einer zementierten Hüftgelenkstotalendoprothese unter Spinalanästhesie – Fallbericht. Anästh Intensivther Notfallmed 24:118–120

Elmaraghy AW, Humeniuk B, Anderson GI, Schemitsch EH, Richards RR (1998) The role of methylmethacrylate monomer in the formation and haemodynamic outcome of pulmonary fat emboli. J Bone Joint Surg Br 80:156–161

Engsæter LB, Strand T, Raugstad TS, Husebo S, Langeland N (1984) Effects of a distal venting hole in the femur during total hip replacement. Arch Orthop Trauma Surg 103:328–331

Eriksson BI, Ekman S, Lindbratt S, Baur M, Bach D, Tørholm C, Kälebo P, Close P (1997) Prevention of thromboembolism with use of recombinant hirudin. J Bone Joint Surg Am 79:326–333

Evans FG, King AI (1961) Regional differences in some physical properties of human spongy bone. In: Evans FG (ed) Biomechanical studies of the musculo-sceletal system. Thomas, Springfield, pp 49–67

Evarts CM, Feil EJ (1971) Prevention of thromboembolic disease after elective surgery of the hip. J Bone Joint Surg Am 53:1271–1280

Eyerer P, Jin R (1986) Influence of mixing technique on some properties of PMMA bone cement. J Biomed Mater Res 20:1057–1094

Francis CW, Marder VJ, Evarts CM (1986) Lower risk of thromboembolic disease after total hip replacement with non-cemented than with cemented prostheses. Lancet :769–771

Fredin HO, Nillius AS (1982) Fatal pulmonary embolism after total hip replacement. Acta Orthop Scand 53:407–411

Fredin HO, Rosberg B (1986) Anaesthetic techniques and thromboembolism in total hip arthroplasty. Eur J Anaesthesiol 3:273–281

Freeman MAR, Cameron HU, Brown GC (1978) Cemented double cup arthroplasty of the hip: a 5 year experience with the ICLH prosthesis. Clin Orthop 134:45–52

Frost HM (1973) Orthopaedic Biomechanics. Thomas, Springfield

Frost HM (1983) A determinant of bone architecture. The minimum effective strain. Clin Orthop 175:286–292

Frost HM (1987) Bone "mass" and the "mechanostat": a proposal. Anat Rec 219:1–9

Gerard Y (1978) Hip arthroplasty by matching cups. Clin Orthop 134:25–35

Gluck T (1891) Autoplastik – Transplantation – Implantation von Fremdkörpern. Verh Berl Med Ges XXI, VIII:79–98

Goldstein SA (1987) The mechanical properties of trabecular bone: dependence on anatomic location and function. J Biomech 20:1055–1061

Goldstein SA, Wilson DL, Sonstegard DA, Matthews LS (1983) The mechanical properties of human tibial trabecular bone as a function of metaphyseal location. J Biomech 16:965–969

Goldstein SA, Matthews LS (1991) The response of trabecular bone to implant load. Orthop Rel Sci 2:185–190

Goodman SB, Schatzker J, Summer-Smith G, et al (1985) The effect of the polymethylmethacrylate on bone: an experimental study. Arch Orthop Traumat Surg 104:150–154

Goodman SB, Huie P, Song Z, Lee K, Doshi A, Rushdieh B, Woolson S, Maloney W, Schurman D, Sibley R (1997) Loosening and osteolysis of cemented joint arthroplasties. Clin Orthop 337:149–163

Gresham GA, Kuczynski A, Rosborough D (1971) Fatal fat embolism following replacement arthroplasty for transcervical fractures of femur. BMJ 2:617–619

Griffith MJ, Seidenstein MK, Williams D, Charnley J (1978) Eight year results of Charnley arthroplasties of the hip with special reference to the behavior of cement. Clin Orthop 137:24–36

Haas SS, Brauer GM, Dixon G (1975) A characterization of polymethyl-methacrylate bone cement. J Bone Joint Surg Am 57:380

Haboush (1953) A new operation for arthroplasty of the hip based on biomechanics, photoelasticity, fast setting dental acrylic and other considerations. Bull Hosp Jt Dis NY 14:242–277

Haddad FS, Cobb AG, Bentley G, Levell NJ, Dowd PM (1996) Hypersensitivity in aseptic loosening of total hip replacements. J Bone Joint Surg Br 78:546–549

Haddad RJ, Cook SD, Thomas KA, Andersen RC, Edmunds JO (1986) Histologic and microradiographic analysis of non-cemented retrieved PCA knee components. In: Abstracts of the 53rd Annual Meeting American Academy of Orthopaedic Surgeons, New Orleans, p 41

Halawa M, Lee AJC, Ling RSM, Vangala SS (1978) The shear strenght of trabecular bone from the femur, and some factors affecting the shear strenght of the cement-bone interface. Arch Orthop Traum Surg 92:19–30

Hallin G, Modig J, Nordgren L, Olerud S (1974) The intramedullary pressure during bone trauma of total hip replacement surgery. J Med Sci 79:51–54

Hamilton HW, Joyce M (1986) Long-term results of low friction arthroplasty performed in a community hospital, including a radiologic review. Clin Orthop 211:55–64

Harris WH (1980) Advances in surgical technique for total hip replacement. Without and with osteotomy of the greater trochanter. Clin Orthop 146:188–204

Harris WH, McGann WA (1986) Loosening of the femoral component after use of the medullary-plug cementing technique. Follow-up note with a minimum five-year follow-up. J Bone Joint Surg Am 68:1064–1066

Harris WH, McKusick K, Athanasoulis CA, Waltman AC, Strauss HW (1984) Detection of pulmonary emboli after total hip replacement using serial $C^{15}O_2$ pulmonary scans. J Bone Joint Surg Am 66:1388–1393

Hastings GW, Mahmud FA (1988) Electrical effects in bone. J Biomed Eng 10:515–521

Hastings GW, Mahmud FA, Martini M (1989) Non-contacting electrode system for the measurement of strain generated potentials in bone. J Biomed Eng 11:403–408

Hayes WC, Carter DR (1976) Post-yield behavior of subchondral trabecular bone. J Biomed Mater Res Symp 7:537–544

Hayes WC, Black D (1979) Post-yield energy absorption characteristics of trabecular bone. In: Buskirk van WC (ed) Biomechanics symposium. American Society of Mechanical Engineers, New York, pp 177–180

Head WC (1981) Wagner surface replacement arthroplasty of the hip – analysis of fourteen failures in forty-one hips. J Bone Joint Surg Am 63:420–427

Heine B (1836) Über die Wiedererzeugung neuer Knochenmasse und Bildung neuer Knochen. Grafes Walthers J Chir 24

Herberts P, Ahnfeldt L, Malchau H, Strömberg C, Andersson GBJ (1989) Multicenter trials and their value in assessing total joint arthroplasty. Clin Orthop 249:48–55

Hochmeister M, Fellinger E, Denk W, Laufer G (1987) Intraoperative tödliche Fett- und Knochenmarksembolie der Lunge bei Implantation einer Hüftendoprothese mit Polymethylmethacrylathaltigem Knochenzement. Z Orthop 125:337–339

Hoffmann CW (1990) Twenty years of total hip arthroplasty in Taranaki – a survival analysis. J Bone Joint Surg Br 73 [Suppl]:23

Hoy ALS, Bloebaum RD, Clarke IC, Sarmiento A (1984) The dynamic bone response to acrylic implantation. Presented at the 30th Annual ORS, Atlanta, Georgia, 7–9 February

Huiskes R, Strens PHGE, Heck van J, Slooff TJJH (1985) Interface stresses in the resurface hip – finite element analysis of load. Acta Orthop Scand 56:474–478

Hukkanen M, Corbett SA, Batten J, Konttinen YT, McCarthy ID, Maclouf J, Santavirta S, Hughes SPF, Polak JM (1997) Aseptic loosening of total hip replacement. J Bone Joint Surg Br 79:467–474

Hvid I, Christensen P, Soondergaard J, Christensen PB, Larsen CG (1983) Compressive strength of tibial cancellous bone. Instron and osteopenetrometer measurements in an autopsy material. Acta Orthop Scand 54:819–825

Hvid I, Jensen J (1984) Cancellous bone strenght at the proximal human tibia. Eng Med 13:21–25

Hyderally H, Miller R (1976) Hypotension and cardiac arrest during prosthetic hip surgery with acrylic bone cement. Ortho Rev 5:55–61

Hyland J, Robins RHS (1970) Cardiac arrest and bone cement. BMJ 4:176–177

Indong OH, Carlson CE, Tomford WW, Harris WH (1978) Improved fixation of the femoral component after total hip replacement using a methacrylate intramedullary plug. J Bone Joint Surg Am 60:608–613

Issendorff WD von, Ritter G (1977) Untersuchungen zur Höhe und Bedeutung des intramedullären Druckes während des Einzementierens von Hüftendoprothesen. Unfallchirurgie 3:99–104

Jasty M, Maloney WJ, Bragdon CR, Haire T, Harris WH (1990) Histomorphological studies of the long-term skeletal responses to well fixed cemented femoral components. J Bone Joint Surg Am 72:1220–1229

Johnson R, Green JR, Charnley J (1977) Pulmonary embolism and its prophylaxis following the charnley total hip replacement. Clin Orthop 127:123–132

Johnson R, Carmichael JHE, Almond HGA, Loynes RP (1978) Deep venous thrombosis following charnley arthroplasty. Clin Orthop 132:24–30

Jolley MN, Salvati EA, Brown GC (1982) Early results and complications of surface replacement of the hip. J Bone Joint Surg Am 64:366–377

Jones RH (1975) Physiologic emboli changes oberved during total hip replacement arthroplasty. Clin Orthop 112:192–200

Jones LC, Hungerford DS (1987) Cement disease. Clin Orthop 225:192–206

Judet J, Judet R (1950) The use of an artificial femoral head for arthroplasty of the hip joint. J Bone Joint Surg Br 32:166

Kafka V (1983) On hydraulic strengthening of bones. Biorheology 20:789–793

Kakkar VV, Bentley PG, Lawrence D, DeHaas HA, Ward VP (1979) Die Prophylaxe der postoperativen, venösen Thromboembolie beim Hüftgelenksersatz mit Heparin und Dihydroergotamin. Munch Med Wochenschr 121:1152–1155

Kakkar VV, Fok PJ, Murray WJ, Paes T, Merenstein D, Dodds R, Farrell R, Crellin RQ, Thomas EM, Morley TR (1985) Heparin and dihydroergotamine prophylaxis against thrombo-embolism after hip arthroplasty. J Bone Joint Surg 67:538–542

Kallos T, Enis JE, Gollan F, Davis JH (1974) Intramedullary pressure and pulmonary embolism of femoral medullary contents in dogs during insertion of bone cements and a prosthesis. J Bone Joint Surg Am 56:1363–1367

Kaplan EL, Meier P (1958) Non-parametric estimation from incomplete observation. J Am Stat Assoc 53:457

Kärrholm J, Hansson LI, Laurin S, Selvik G (1982) Roentgen stereophotogrammetric study of growth pattern after fracture through tibial shaft, ankle and heel. Case report. Arch Orthop Traumat Surg 99:253–258

Kärrholm J, Malchau H, Snorrason F, Herberts P (1994) Micromotion of femoral stems in total hip arthroplasty. J Bone Joint Surg Am 76:1692–1705

Kavanagh BF, Dewity MA, Ilstrup DM, Stauffer RN, Coventry MB (1989) Charnley total hip arthroplasty with cement. J Bone Joint Surg Am 71:1496–1503

Kavanagh BF, et al (1994) Charnley low friction arthroplasty of the hip twenty year results with cement. J Arthroplasty 9:229–234

Keller JC, Lautenschlager EP (1983) Experimental attempts to reduce acrylic porosity. Biomat Med Dev Art Org 11:221–236

Kepes ER, Underwood PS, Becsey L (1972) Intraoperative death associated with acrylic bone cement. JAMA 222:576–578

Kiaer (1953) Preliminary report on arthroplasty by use of acrylic head. Cinquieme congres international de chirurgie orthopedique, Stockholm 1951. Lielene, Brussels

Kleinschmidt O (1941) Plexiglas zur Deckung von Schädellücken. Chirurg 13:273

Kobayashi S, Eftekhar NS, Terayama K (1996) Long term bone remodeling around the Charnley femoral prostheses. Clin Orthop 326:162–173

König F (1913) Über die Implantation von Elfenbein zum Ersatz von Knochen- und Gelenkenden. Beitr Klin Chir 85:91–114

Krause WR, Krug B, Miller J (1982) Strength of the cement-bone interface. Clin Orthop 163:290–299

Kummer B (1963) Grundlagen der Biomechanik des menschlichen Stütz-und Bewegungsapparates. IX Congr Internat Chir Orthopaed Traumatol II. Med Akademie, Vienna, pp 65–88

Lanyon LE (1973) Analysis of surface bone strain in the calcaneus of sheep during normal locomotion. J Biomech 6:41

Lazcano MA, Campos Aceves LF, Sauri Arce JC (1995) Charnley low friction arthroplasty – a 20 to 25 year follow-up and study of the failures in patients younger than 65 years. In: ACORA (ed) Charnley total hip arthroplasty. Transit Communications, Lyon

Lee AJC, Ling RSM, Wrighton JD (1973) Some properties of polymethyl-methacrylate with reference to its use in orthopaedic surgery. Clin Orthop 95:281

Lee AJC, Ling RSM (1981) Improved cemented techniques. In: Murray DG (ed) Instructional course lectures, vol XXX. Mosby, St. Louis, pp 407–413

Lewalle J, Akalay A, Bertrand M, et al (1995) 20 year follow up of Charnley L.F.A.: What could it still teach us? In: ACORA (ed) Charnley total hip arthroplasty. Transit Communications, Lyon

Lidgren L, Bodelind B, Möller J (1984) Bone cement improved by vacuum mixing and chilling. Acta Orthop Scand 57:27–32

Liedloff H, Brauckhoff KF, Heerdegen R, Barthel W (1984) Zur Anwendung von Heparin in Kombination mit Dihydroergotamin zur postoperativen Thromboseprophylaxe bei Hüftgelenkoperationen. Z Ges Inn Med 39:428–431

Liedloff H, Brauckhoff KF (1989) Medikamentöse Thromboembolieprophylaxe in der elektiven Hüftchirurgie unter Berücksichtigung thrombophiler Zustände. Z Ges Inn Med 44:320–323

Linde F, Hvid I, Jensen NC (1985) Material properties of cancellous bone in repetitive axial loading. Eng Med 14:173–177

Linde F, Hvid I (1989) The effect of constraint on the mechanical behavior of trabecular bone specimens. J Biomech 22:485–490

Linde F, Pongsoipetch B, Frich LH, Hvid I (1990) Three-axial strain controlled testing applied to bone specimens from the proximal tibial epiphysis. J Biomech 23:1167–1172

Linder L, Hansson HA (1983) Ultrastructural aspects of the interface between bone and cement in man. Report of three cases. J Bone Joint Surg Br 65:646–649

Lindstrand A, Selvik G (1976) A stereophotogrammetric analysis of the interior drawer sign in acute lateral ligament ruptures of the ankle joint. In: Lindstrand A (ed) Lateral lesions in sprained ankles. Thesis, University of Lund

Ling RSM (1981) Loosening experiences at Exeter. Orthop Trans 5:351

Lotke PA, Palevsky H, Keenan AM, Meranze S, Steinberg ME, Ecker ML, Kelley MA (1996) Aspirin and Warfarin for thromboembolic disease after total joint arthroplasty. Clin Orthop 324:251–258

Madey SM, Callaghan JJ, Olejniczak JP, et al (1997) Charnley total hip arthroplasty with use of improved techniques of cementing. J Bone Joint Surg Am 79:53–64

Malcolm AJ (1990) Pathology of cemented low-friction arthroplasties in autopsy-specimens. In: Older O (ed) Implant bone interface. Springer, Berlin Heidelberg New York, pp 77–82

Malchau H, Herberts P, Ahnfeldt L (1993) Prognosis of total hip replacement in Sweden. Follow-up of 92.675 operations performed 1978–1990. Acta Orthop Scand 64:497–506

Malchau H, Herberts P (1996) Prognosis of total hip replacement. Surgical and cementing technique in THR: a revision-risk study of 134,056 primary operations. Presented at 63rd Annual Meeting of the American Academy of Orthopaedic Surgeons, 22–26 February 1996, Atlanta

Malcolm AJ (1990) Pathology of cemented low-friction arthroplasties in autopsy-specimens. In: Older J (ed) Implant bone interface. Springer, Berlin Heidelberg New York, pp 77–82

Maloney WJ, Sychterz C, Bragdon C et al (1996) Skeletal response to well fixed femoral components inserted with and without cement. Clin Orthop 33:15–26

Markolf KL, Amstutz HC (1976a) In vitro measurement of bone-acrylics interface pressure during femoral component insertion. Clin Orthop 121:60–66

Markolf KL, Amstutz HC (1976b) Penetration and flow of acrylic bone cement. Clon Orthop 121: 99–102

Maxeiner H (1988) Tödliche, intraoperative Lungenfettembolie bei Endoprothese des Hüftgelenkes. Beitr Gerichtl Med 47:415–427

McElhaney JH (1966) Dynamic response of bone and muscle tissue. J Appl Physiol 21:1231–1236

McKee GK, Watson-Farrar J (1965) Prosthetic replacement of arthritic hips by means of the McKee-Farrar artificial hip joint. J Bone Joint Surg Br 47:185

McKee GK, Watson-Farrar J (1966) Replacement of arthritic hips by the McKee-Farrar prosthesis. J Bone Joint Surg Br 48:245–259

McKee GK, Watson-Farrar J (1970) Development of total prosthetic replacement of the hip. Clin Orthop 72:85

Merkel F (1874) Betrachtung über das Os femoralis. Arch Path Anat LIX (2):237–256

Michelinakis E, Morgan RH, Curtis PJ (1971) Circulatory arrest and bone cement. BMJ 3:639

Miller EH, Serot DI (1978) Breathing zone concentration of the monomer of methylmethacrylate during total hip replacement operations. The Hip Society. Proceedings of the Fourth Open Scientific Meeting. Mosby, St. Louis, pp 260–263.

Milne IS (1973) Hazards of acrylic bone cement – a report of two cases. Anaesthesia 28:538–543

Mjöberg B, Hansson LI, Selvik G (1984) Instability of total hip prosthesis at rotational stress. A roentgen stereophotogrammetric study. Acta Orthop Scand 55:504–506

Modig J, Borg T, Karlström G, Maripuu E, Sahlstedt B (1983) Thromboembolism after total hip replacement: role of epidural and general anesthesia. Anesth Analg 62:174–180

Mogensen B, Ekelund L, Hansson LI, Lidgren L, Selvik G (1982) Surface replacements in the hip in chronic arthritis. A clinical radiographic and roentgen stereophotogrammetric evaluation. Acta Orthop Scand 53:929–936

Montrey JS, Kistner RL, Kong AYT, Lindberg RF, Mayfield GW, Jones DA, Mitsunaga MM (1985) Thromboembolism following hip fracture. J Trauma 25:534–537

Moore AT (1957) The self-locking metal hip prosthesis. J Bone Joint Surg Am 39:811–827

Müller ME (1975) Total hip replacement: planning, technique and complications. In: Cruess and Mitchell (eds) Surgical management of degenerative arthritis of the lower limb. Lea and Febiger, Philadelphia

Müller ME, Ellmiger B (1979) Coxarthrose. 10-Jahresergebnisse der sogenannten Setzholz-Totalprothese. Orthopäde 8:73

Neumann L, Freund KG, Sörenson KH (1994) Long-term results of Charnley total hip replacement. Review of 92 patients at 15 to 20 years. J Bone Joint Surg Br 76:245–251

Newens AF, Volz RG (1972) Severe hypotension during prosthetic hip surgery with acrylic bone cement. Anesthesiology 36:298–300

Nice EJM (1973) Case report: cardiac arrest following use of acrylic bone cement. Anaesth Intens Care 1:244–245

Nillius AS, Nylander G (1979) Deep vein thrombosis after total hip replacement: a clinical and phlebographic study. Br J Surg 66:324–326

Nilsen DTW, Naess-Andresen KF, Kierulf P, Heldaas J, Stören G, Godal HC (1984) Graded pressure stockings in prevention of deep vein thrombosis following total hip replacement. Acta Chir Scand 150:531–534

Noble PC, Alexander JW, Lindahl LJ, Yew DT, Granberry WM, Tullos HS (1988) The anatomic basis of femoral component design. Clin Orthop 235:148–165

Oh I, Charlson CE, Tomford WW, Harris WH (1978) Improved fixation of the femoral component after total hip replacement using a methacrylate intramedullary plug. J Bone Joint Surg Am 60:608–613

Ohnsorge P (1971) Experimentelle Untersuchungen zur Bestimmung des intramedullären Druckverlaufes im Femur beim Eindrücken von Knochenzement und beim Einbringen einer Femurschaftendoprothese. Thesis, University of Cologne

Older J (1986) Low-friction arthroplasty of the hip. A 10–12-year follow-up study. Clin Orthop Rel Res 211:36–42

Older J (1995) The Charnley LFA at 25 years with a worldwide review. In: Caton J, Michel F and Picault C (eds) Charnley total hip arthroplasty. ACORA, Lyon, pp 25–29

Olsson TH, Selvik G, Willner S (1976) Kinematic analysis of spinal fusion. Invest Radiol 11:202–209

Orsini EC, Byrick RJ, Mullen JBM, Kay JC, Waddell JP (1987) Cardiopulmonary function and pulmonary microemboli during arthroplasty using cemented or non-cemented components: the role of intramedullary pressure. J Bone Joint Surg Am 69:822–832

Patterson BM, Healey JH, Cornell CN, Sharrock NE (1991) Cardiac arrest during hip arthroplasty with a cemented long stem component. J Bone Joint Surg Am 73:271–277

Pauwels F (1965) Gesammelte Abhandlungen zur funktionellen Anatomie des Bewegungsapparates. Springer, Berlin Heidelberg New York

Peebles DJ, Ellis RH, Stride SDK, Simpson BRJ (1972) Cardiovascular effects of methylmethacrylate cement. BMJ 1:349–351

Pellegrini jr VD, Clement D, Lush-Ehmann C, Keller GS, McCollister Evarts C (1996) Natural history of hromboembolic disease after total hip arthroplasty. Clin Orthop 333:27–40

Perren S, Cordey J (1977) Die Gewebsdifferenzierung in der Frakturheilung. Z Unfallheilk 80:161

Petersen H (1927) Über den Feinbau der menschlichen Skelettteile. Roux Arch 112:112–137

Phillips H, Cole PV, Lettin AWF (1971) Cardiovascular effects of implanted acrylic bone cement. BMJ 3:460–461

Phillips H, Lettin AWF, Cole PV (1973) Cardiovascular effects of implanted acrylic cement. J Bone Joint Surg Br 55:210

Pitto RP, Kössler M, Draenert K (1998) Prophylaxis of fat and bone marrow embolism in cemented total hip arthroplasty. Clin Orthop 355: 23–34

Powell JN, McGrath PJ, Lahiri SK, Hill P (1970) Cardiac arrest associated with bone cement. BMJ 3:326

Radin EL, Paul IL, Tolkoff JT (1970) Subchondral bone changes in patients with early degenerative joint disease. Arthr Rheum 13:400–405

Rahn BA, Perren SM (1971) Xylenol Orange, a fluorochrome useful in polychrome sequential labeling of calcifying tissues. Stain Technol 46:125–129

Ritter MA, Gioe TJ (1986) Conventional versus resurfacing total hip arthroplasty. J Bone Joint Surg Am 68:216–225

Röttger J, Elson R (1986) A modification of Charnley low-friction arthroplasty. Representative ten-year follow-up results of the St. Georg prosthesis. Clin Orthop 211:154–163

Rubin CT, Lanyon IE (1987) Osteoregulatory nature of mechanical stimuli: function as a determinant for adaptive remodelling in bone. J Orthop Res 5:300–310

Ruckelshausen MC (1964) Mechanisch-technische Probleme der Hüft-Alloplastik. Z Orthop 99:46–56

Rüegsegger P, Anliker M, Drambacher M (1982) Quantification of trabecular bone with low dose computer tomography. J Comput Assist Tomogr 5:384

Russe W (1988) Röntgenkontrastphotogrammetrie der künstlichen Hüftgelenkspfanne. Huber, Bern

Russotti GM, Coventry MB, Stauffer RN (1988) Cemented total hip arthroplasty with contemporary techniques. A five-year minimum follow-up study. Clin Orthop 235:141–147

Ryd L, Boegard T, Egund N, et al (1983) Migration of the tibial component in successful unicompartment knee arthroplasty. A clinical, radiographic and roentgen stereophotogrammetric study. Acta Orthop Scand 54:408–416

Ryd L (1986) Micromotion in knee arthroplasty. A roentgen stereophotogrammetric analysis of tibial component fixation. Acta Orthop Scand [Suppl 220]:57

Salvati EA, Wilson PD (1973) Long-term results of femoral-head replacement. J Bone Joint Surg Am 55:516–524

Salvati EA, Im VC, Aglietti P, Wilson PD Jr (1976) Radiology of total hip replacements. Clin Orthop 121:74–82

Salvati EA, Wilson jr PD, Jolley NM, Vakili F, Aglietti P, Brown GC (1981) A ten-year follow-up study of our first one hundred consecutive Charnley total hip replacements. J Bone Joint Surg Am 63:753–767

Salzer M, Knahr K, Locke H, Stärk N (1978) Cement-free bioceramic double-cup endoprosthesis of the hip-joint. Clin Orthop 134:80–86

Schlag G (1974) Experimentelle und klinische Untersuchungen mit Knochenzementen. Ein Beitrag zur Pathogenese und Prophylaxe der akuten intraoperativen Hypotension bei Hüftalloarthroplastiken. Hollinek, Vienna

Schlag G, Schliep HJ, Dingeldein E, Grieben A, Ringsdorf W (1976) Sind intraoperative Kreislaufkomplikationen bei Alloarthroplastiken des Hüftgelenkes durch Methylmetacylat bedingt? Anaesthesist 25:60–67

Schmidt J (1996) Das transprothetische Drainagesystem zur optimierten Zementierung von Hüftendoporthesenschäften. Operat Orthop Traumatol 3:239–242

Schreiber A, Jacob HAC (1984) Loosening of the femoral component of the ICLH double cup hip prosthesis – a biomechanical investigation with reference to clinical results. Acta Orthop Scand [Suppl 207]

Schulitz KP, Koch H, Dustmann HO (1971) Lebensbedrohliche Sofortkomplikationen durch Fettembolie nach Einsetzen von Totalendoprothesen mit Polymethylmethacrylat. Arch Orthop Unfall Chir 71:307–315

Schulte KR, Callaghan JJ, Kelley SS, Johnston RC (1993) The outcome of Charnley total hip arthroplasty with cement after a minimum twenty-year follow up. J Bone Joint Surg Am 75:961–975

Scott GC, Korostoff E (1990) Oscillatory and step response electromechanical phenomena in human and bovine bone. J Biomech 23:127–143

Seelig W, Ludin U, Morscher E (1989) Perioperative Risiken und Probleme beim Totalhüftgelenksersatz. Schweiz Rundsch Med Prax 4:390–393

Selvik G (1974) A roentgen stereophotogrammetric method for the study of the kinematics of the skeletal system. Thesis, University of Lund

Selvik G, Hansson Li, Landstrand A, Mjöberg B, Ryd L (1985) Roentgen stereophotogrammetric analysis (RSA) in total hip and knee joint replacement. In: Whittle M, Harris D (eds) Biomechanical measurements in orthopaedic practice. Oxford University Press, Oxford

Sevitt S (1972) Fat embolism in patients with fractured hips. BMJ 2:257–262

Shao WR, Foster T, Leland RH, Bachus KN (1993) Atrophy of cancellous bone due to microcasting. 39th Annual Meeting Orthop Research Society San Francisco, Feb 15–18

Sherman RMP, Byrick RJ, Kay JC, Sullivan TR, Waddell JP (1983) The role of lavage in preventing haemodynamic and blood-gas changes during cemented arthroplasty. J Bone Joint Surg Am 65:500–506

Siebler G, Edler S, Kuner EH (1988) Zur Totalendoprothese bei der Schenkelhalsfraktur des alten Menschen – eine Analyse von 284 Fällen. Unfallchirurg 91:291–298

Slooff TJ (1971) The influence of acrylic cement. An experimental study. Acta Orthop Scand 42:465–481

Slooff TJ (1972) Experiments with acrylic cement. In: Orthopaedic Surgery and Traumatology. Proceedings of the 12th Congress of the SICOT, Tel Aviv, 9–12 October 1972. Excerpta Medica, Amsterdam

Smith RE, Turner RJ (1973) Total hip replacement using methylmethacrylate cement. Clin Orthop 95:231–238

Smith-Petersen MN (1948) Evolution of mould arthroplasty of the hip joint. J Bone Joint Surg Br 30:59–75

Soltesz U, Ege W (1992) Fatigue behavior of different acrylic bone cements. Presented at the Fourth World Biomaterials Congress, Berlin

Stamatakis JD, Sagar S, Maffei H, Lawrence D, Kakkar VV (1976) Femoral vein thrombosis and total hip replacement arthroplasty. Br J Surg 63:668–669

Stamatakis JD, Kakkar VV, Sagar S, Lawrence D, Nairn D, Bentley PG (1977) Femoral vein thrombosis and total hip replacement. BMJ 2:223–225

Stauffer RN (1982) Ten-year follow-up study of total hip replacement. J Bone Joint Surg Am 64:983–990

Sutherland CJ, Wilde AH, Borden LS, Marks KE (1982) A ten-year follow-up of hundred consecutive Müller curved-stem total hip-replacement arthroplasties. J Bone Joint Surg Am 64:970–982

Sychterz CJ, Engh CA (1996) The influence of clinical factors on periprosthetic bone remodeling. Clin Orthop 322:285–292

Tanaka S (1978) Surface replacement of the hip joint. Clin Orthop 134:75–79

Terayama K (1986) Experience with Charnley low-friction arthroplasty in Japan. Clin Orthop 211:79–84

Thomas TA, Sutherland IC, Waterhouse TD (1971) Cold curing acrylic bone cement: a clinical study of the cardiovascular side effects during hip joint replacement. Anaesthesia 26:298–303

Thompson FR (1954) Two and a half year's experience with a vitallium intramedullary hip prosthesis. J Bone Joint Surg Am 36:489–502

Thorburn J, Louden JR, Vallance R (1980) Spinal and general anaesthesia in total hip replacement: frequency of deep vein thrombosis. Br J Anaesth 52:1117–1121

Tillmann B (1981) Funktionelle Morphologie des menschlichen Hüftgelenks. Histo-Morphologie des Bewegungsapparates 1:141–152

Tillmann K, Thabe H (1983) Gelenkflächenersatz bei rheumatischer Coxitis. Med Orthop Techn 103:103–120

Tjörnstrand B, Selvik G, Egund N, Lindstrand A (1981) Roentgen stereophotogrammetric analysis in high tibial osteotomy for gonarthrosis. Arch Orthop Traumat Surg 99: 73–81

Tronzo RG, Kallos T, Wyche MQ (1974) Elevation of intramedullary pressure when methylmethacrylate is inserted in total hip arthroplasty. J Bone Joint Surg 56 a: 714–718

Tscherne H, Westermann K, Trentz O, Pretschner P, Mellmann J (1978) Thromboembolische Komplikationen und ihre Prohylaxe beim Hüftgelenkersatz. Unfallheilkunde 81:178–187

Turner CH (1989) Yield behavior of bovine cancellous bone. J Biomech Eng 111:256–260

Ulrich C (1995) Stellenwert der Entlastungsbohrung zur Reduzierung der Knochenmarksausschüttung bei zementierten Hüftendoprothesen. Orthopädie 24: 138–144

Ulrich C, Burri C, Wörsdörfer O, Heinrich H (1986) Intraoperative transoesophageale two-dimensional echocardiography in total hip replacement. Arch Orthop Trauma Surg 105:274–278

Ulrich C, Wörsdorfer O, Heinrich C (1985) Intraoperative transoesophageale zweidimensionale Echokardiographie bei Hüftprothesenimplantaten. In: Draenert K (Ed) Die Implantatverankerung. Symosien in Orthopädie und Chirurgie des Bewegungsapparates, p 35–36, Munich: Art and Science

Van Der Vis HM, Aspenberg P, Marti RK, Tigchelaar W, Van Noorden CJF (1998) Fluid pressure causes bone resorption in a rabbit model of prosthetic loosening. Clin Orthop 350:201–208

Wagner H (1978) Surface replacement of the hip. Clin Orthop 134:102–130

Walker TW, Graham JD, Mills RH (1976) Changes in the mechanical behavior of the human femoral heads associated with arthritic pathologies. J Biomech 9:615–624

Weidenreich F (1922) Über die Beziehung zwischen Muskelapparat und Knochen und dem Charakter des Knochengewebes. Anat Anz 55:28–53

Weinstein AM, Bingham DN, Sauer BW, Lunceford EM (1976) The effect of high pressure insertion and antibiotic inclusions upon the mechanical properties of polymethylmethacrylate. Clin Orthop 121:67–73

Wenda K, Issendorff WD von, Rudigier J, Ritter G (1988) Der Einfluss des Markraumsperrers auf den intramedullären Druck während Prothesenimplantationen. Hefte zur Unfallheilkunde, Heft 200:5. Deutsch-Österreichisch-Schweizerische Unfalltagung. Berlin-Heidelberg-New York: Springer-Verlag

Wille-Jörgensen P, Winter-Christensen S, Bjerg-Nielsen A, Stadeager C, Kjær L (1989) Prevention of Thromboembolism following elective hip surgery. Clin Orthop 247:163–167

Wroblewski BM (1986) 15–21-year results of the Charnley low-friction arthroplasty. Clin Orthop 211:30–35

Wroblewski BM (1990) Charnley low-friction arthroplasty: a study of results in young patients. J Bone Joint Surg Br 73:71

Wroblewski BM, Sidney PD (1993) Charnley low friction arthroplasty of the hip. Long term results. Clin Orthop 292:191–201

Wroblewski BM, Taylor GW, Siney P (1992) Charnley low-friction arthroplasty: 19-to-25 year results. Orthopedics 15:421–424

Zichner L (1987) Embolien aus dem Knochenmarkskanal nach Einsetzen von intramedullären Femurkopfendoprothesen mit Polymethylmethacrylat. Aktuel Probl Chir Orthop 31:201–205

Zippel H (1990) Multimorbidität und perioperatives Risiko der Hüftgelenktotalendoprothetik (HTEP). Beitr Orthop Traumatol 37:193–203

ZOW-Report (1998) Manual der Zementiertechnik, ZOW Munich

Subject Index

Acetabular roof **38 f, 41 f**
Acetabulum 2, **38 ff**, 86
    Preparatory steps **39**
    Exposure of the acetabulum **39**
    Fossa acetabuli **40**
    Preparation of the bony acetabulum **40**
    Joint surface **41**
    Inclination and alignment **42**
Alignment 41, **42** f, 55 f, 84 f, **86**
    Posterior tangential alignment 55 f
Anchorage 2-6, **14 ff, 38**, 83, 97
    Bony anchorage 15 f
    Distal anchorage 16 f
    Proximal anchorage 14 ff
Anisotropy 22, 25
Anterolateral approach **34 f**
Anticoagulation **41** f
Approach to the hip **34 ff**, 55
    Posterolateral approach **34**
    Transgluteal approach **36**
Atrophy 14, **28 f**, 32, 97-98

Biomechanics **19 ff**
    E-modulus **20-22**, 26
    Elasticity **19** f
    Viscoelasticity **20**
    Isotropic deformation **20**
    Resilience and damping **20** f
    Compliance **22**
    Energy **22**
    Impact **22**
Blood coagulate **33**
Bone
    -atrophy 28
    -density 22, **24,** 26
    -healing **24**
    -lamellar 29
    -rasp 33
    -remodeling **22** f
Bone cement 3, 6, **7 ff, 14 ff, 26 ff,45 ff, 70 ff**
    Bone cement application **53 ff**
    Bone cement implants **7**ff
    TCP bone cement **11**ff
    HA bone cement **11** ff
    Preparation of the bone cement **45 ff**
Bone cement polymerization **48** f
Bone-to-cement contact **4, 7 ff, 26** f
Bone-to-cement interface 6, 11, **27**
Bone-to-implant interface **19** f
Breaking strength **21** ff
Buchholz prosthesis **5**

Calcar femoris 17, 33, 79 f, **81 ff**, 86, 92
Cardiovascular incident 4, 72
Cartilage **40**
Cementation **70** f, **96** ff
Cement disease **4**
Cement interface **29**
Cemented press-fit **16** f

Cementing technique 13, 30, **41 ff, 53 ff, 69-71**
Centralizing **85**
Charnley, John **3**
Charnley prosthesis 4, 5
Compact bone **19**
Compliance **22**, 24,
Connective tissue 6, 11, 28
Cyclic loads **22**

Damping **20 ff**
Deformation **20 ff**, 96
Diamond instrumentation 33, 39, 40, **55, 57 ff**, 86
    Diamond cutting tool **55** ff
Diaphyseal hypertrophy 6
Drainage **61** ff, **72** ff
Drill hole **76** f
Drill jig **61**

Elasticity **19 ff**
E-modulus **20-22**, 26
Embolism **67**
Energy **22,** 24
Epiphyseal spongiosa **29**
Epiphysis of the femur **30 ff**

Fascia lata **34**
Fatal incidence **72-74**
Fibrous tissue 9, **14 ff**, 22, 24
Filler material **11 ff**
Fluorescence 28, 86
Fossa acetabuli **40**
Fracture 5, 26, 28

Gap healing **8**, 24, 26-27, 30-31, 98
Gentamicin 11, 48-50
Giant cells 6

Haversian system 9, 19
HDPE cup **28**
Hematoma **8**
Heparin **70**, 76
Histomorphology **24, 28 ff**, 86
Histomorphology of human samples **14 ff**
Homogeneous mixture **47 ff**
Hook's law **20**
Hydroxyapatite (HA) 6, **11 ff**, 24, 50

Iliac vein **4**
Impact **22**
Implant 2, **22 ff**, 24, **55 ff, 65 ff**, 70 f, 86
    Deformation **22** ff
    Implantation axis **55 ff**
    Implant-surface **22 ff**
Implant's bed (preparation) **65 ff**
Inclination **42** f
Infection **4**
Instrumentation **94 ff**
    Medullary cavity plug **68**
    Plug applicator **69**

Subject Index

Rasp **59 f**
Tissue protector **61 f**
Troicar **63**
Interlocking of the prosthesis 67 f, 82, 96-98
Isotropic deformation **20**
Isthmus of the femur **86**

Jet lavage 33, 41, 67
Joint surface **41**

Lavage **41 f**, **67**, 76, 96-97
Linea aspera **75 ff**
Loosening 4-6, **15**, 28, 96
    Overall loosening 4
Loosening, definitive 5
Loosening, probable **6**
Low friction arthroplasty 5
Low viscosity bone cement **46 f**, 97
Luxation 66

Mechanostat **23**
Medullary canal 7, 8, 14, **55 ff**, **61 ff**, 68, 70, **72 ff**, 86, 92
    Opening **55 ff**
    Drainage **61 ff**, **72 ff**
    Thromboembolism **72 ff**
    Distal drill hole **76 ff**
Medullary cavity plug (MPC) **77**, **68 f**, 97
Miller-Galante-Tibia prosthesis 26-27
Müller prosthesis 5-6, **14 ff**, **55**, 86

Necrosis 2, **30**, 98

Offset **86 f**, 90
Os ischii 41
Os pubis 38, 41
Osteocytes 6, 23-24, **30 ff**
Osteolysis **16**
Osteotomy **39**, 55, 70, 92
    Inclination **39**

Pain 5
Pelvis 38
Periosteal bone renewal 8, 9
Polychromatic sequence marking 30
Polymerization curves **46, 48**
Polymerization of bone cement **47 ff**
Polymethylmethacrylate (PMMA) 2, 6, 11, **45 ff**, 50
    Homogeneous mixture 47 ff
    Low viscosity bone cement 46 ff
    Standard viscosity bone cement 45 ff
    Polymerization 46 ff
Porosity of bone cement **48**
Pre-operative planning **86**, 92
Preparation of the bone cement **45 ff**
Preparation of the femur **55 ff**
Pre-pressurizing **50 ff**, 70
Press-fit **16 f**, 22, 96
Pressure 20, 24, **48 f**, 72, **73**, 97
    Inner pressure 20

Intramedullary pressure 73
Proliferation pressure 20
Vapor pressure 48 f
Prostaglandin E2 23
Prosthesis **83 ff**, 86, **91-92**
    Charnley prosthesis 4-5
    Miller-Galante-Tibia prosthesis 26-27
    Müller Prosthesis 5-6, **14 ff**, **55**, 86
Prosthetic design 6, **79 ff**
Proximal anchorage 14 ff
Pulmonary embolism 4, 72

Radiolucent line 4-5, 18
Radiolucent zone 4-5
Relative motions **22**, 24
Remodeling 15
Resilience **20 ff**
Revascularization **8 ff**, 30, 98
Rotation 79, **81**, 83, 86, 89

Shenton line 83, 86, 92
Socket 6
Spongiosa 22, **25 ff**, 33, 38, 40, 76, **79 f**, 92
Spongiosa framework 24
Spongy bone **19**, 22, 28
Standard viscosity bone cement **45 f**, 70
Stem design **83 ff**, 86, **91-92**
Steri Tray **94**
Stiffening of spongiosa 14, **79 f**
Stiffness of bone 20 ff, 97
Strain **20 ff**, 26
Stress **20 ff**, 26, 96-97
Stress shielding 28, 32

Teflon-covered stirring rod **47**
Tensile strength **21 f**
Thromboembolism 4, 67, **72 ff**, 76
Tissue 4, 6, 9, 14 ff, 22-24, 28, 77, 96
Toughness of bone **21 ff**
Trabeculae **11 ff**, **22 ff**, 25-26, 30 ff, 97
Transgluteal approach **36 f**
Tricalciumphosphate (TCP) 6, **11 ff**, 50

Vacuum technique 13, 30, **41 ff**, **53 ff**, **69-71**
    Artifact-free cement filling 54
    Bubble-free bone cement 53 f
    Medullary plug 69 ff
    Vacuum mixed bone cement 53
Valgisation 83
Van-der-Waal's bonds **20**
Viscoelasticity **20 ff**

Wagner cup 26, **28 f**
Ward's zone 79

X-ray 6, 9, 23, 78, 86

Young's modulus 24, 26

Author Index

Aglietti 3, 4, 5, 103
Ahnfeldt 96, 97, 101, 102
Akalay 96, 102
Alexander 86, 96, 103
Alho 24, 26, 99
Almond 73, 101
Amstutz 67, 68, 96, 97, 99, 102
Andersen 26, 101
Anderson GI 73, 100
Anderson LD 2, 99
Andersson 96, 101
Anliker 26, 103
Aronsson 97, 99
Aspenberg 6, 104
Athanasoulis 72, 101
Aufranc 2, 99

Bach 73, 100
Bachus 97, 104
Balderson 97, 99
Ballard 97, 99
Barthel 72
Barton 2, 99
Batten 6, 101
Bauer 34, 36, 99
Baur 73, 100
Beckenbaugh 4, 5, 6, 74, 96, 99
Becsey 74, 102
Beisaw 73, 99
Bell 28, 99
Benjamin 46, 53, 97, 99
Bentley G 6, 101
Bentley PG 73, 102, 104
Bereiter 81, 99
Bertrand 96, 102
Bingham 97, 104
Bjerg-Nielsen 72, 104
Black 24, 101
Blacker 4, 5, 99
Bloebaum 32, 97, 99, 101
Bodelind 48, 102
Boegard 97, 103
Boerner 98, 99
Bogner 72, 74, 99
Borden 5, 104
Borg 72, 73, 103
Borris 73, 99
Brady 5, 99
Bragdon 6, 97, 101
Brauckhoff 72, 73, 102
Brauer 48, 101
Breed 72, 73, 76, 99
Breusch 23, 24, 98, 99
Brighton 23, 99
Brown AM 3, 99
Brown GC 3, 5, 28, 101, 103
Buchholz 26, 99
Burgess 74, 99
Burri 72, 76, 104

Bylander 97, 99
Byrick 67, 73, 97, 103, 104

Callaghan 96, 97, 99, 102, 104
Cameron 28, 101
Campos Aceves 96, 102
Carlson 73, 101
Carmichael 73, 101
Carter 6, 24, 99, 101
Charlson 68, 97, 103
Charnely 2, 3, 4, 5, 6, 33, 55, 72, 74, 86, 96, 97, 98, 99, 101
Chen 6, 99
Christensen P 26, 101
Christensen PB 26, 101
Christiansen 73, 99
Ciarelli 22, 99
Claes 28, 100
Clarac 96, 100
Clarius 67, 72, 74, 75, 100
Clarke IC 97, 101
Clarke MT 72, 73, 100
Clement 72, 73, 103
Close 73
Cobb 6, 101
Cohen 74, 100
Cole 73, 74, 103
Colwell 6, 99
Comerota 73, 99
Convery 4, 100
Cook 26, 100, 101
Corbett 6, 101
Cordey 24, 103
Cornell 72, 74, 103
Coventry 4, 5, 72, 96, 100, 102, 103
Crawford 4, 99
Crellin 72, 102
Currey 26, 100
Curtis 74, 103

D´Lima 6, 99
Dall 4, 5, 100
Dandy 74, 100
Daniel 72, 100
Davis FM 73, 100
Davis JH 72, 73, 76, 102
DeAngelis 74, 100
Dedrich 78
DeHaas 73, 102
Delling 28, 100
Demarest 48, 100
Denk 74, 101
Dewity 96, 102
Dickie 22, 99
Dingeldein 72, 104
Diserio 73, 99
Dixon 48, 101
Dodds 72, 102
Dorr 72, 100
Doshi 6, 101

Author Index

Dowd 6, 101
Draenert K 6, 7, 8, 11, 23, 24, 25, 26, 38, 41, 57, 69, 72, 76, 77, 79, 86, 92, 96, 97, 98, 99, 100, 103
Draenert Y 23, 24, 25, 26, 38, 57, 77, 79, 86, 92, 96, 97, 98, 99, 100
Drambacher 26, 103
Drinker 73, 100
Dustmann 74, 104

Ecker 73
Edler 72, 104
Edmunds 26, 101
Eftekhar 3, 4, 5, 100, 102
Egbert 74, 100
Ege 52, 104
Egund 97, 99, 103
Ekelund 97, 103
Ekman 73, 100
Ellis 74, 103
Ellmiger 54, 103
Elmaraghy 73, 100
Elson 5, 103
Engelbrecht 28, 100
Engh 24, 104
Engsaeter 73, 74, 100
Enis 72, 73, 76, 102
Eriksson 73, 100
Evans 24, 100
Evarts 73, 100
Eyerer 48, 100

Faiss 28, 100
Farrell 72, 102
Feil 73, 100
Fellinger 74, 101
Flynn 22, 99
Foate 73, 100
Fok 72, 102
Follacci 4, 99
Fornasier 28, 99
Foster 97, 104
Francis 73, 100
Fredin 72, 73, 100
Freeman 28, 101
Freund 96, 103
Frich 23, 102
Frost 19, 20, 23, 24, 26, 101

Gautier 81, 99
Gerard 28, 101
Gerngross 28, 100
Gie 46, 53, 97, 99
Gillespie 73, 100
Gioe 28, 103
Gluck 1, 101
Godal 73
Goel 73, 100
Goldstein 22, 23, 26, 99, 101
Gollan 72, 73, 76, 102
Goodman 6, 28, 32, 97, 99, 101
Gradinger 74, 100
Graham 24, 104
Granberry 86, 96, 103
Green 72, 73, 100, 101
Gregg 72, 73, 100
Gresham 74, 101
Grieben 72, 104
Griffith 4, 5, 101
Grobbelaar 5, 100
Gross 23, 99
Groth 73, 99
Gruen 32, 67, 68, 97, 99
Gunn 4, 100

Haas 48, 101
Haboush 2, 3, 101

Haddad 6, 26, 100, 101
Haire 6, 97, 101
Halawa 67, 97, 101
Hallin 73, 101
Hamilton 5, 101
Hammond 4, 99
Hamsa 2, 99
Hannson 97, 99
Hansen 11
Hansson HA 6, 97, 102
Hansson LJ 97, 99, 102, 103, 104
Harper 72, 73, 100
Harris 4, 5, 6, 68, 72, 73, 97, 98, 101, 103
Hastings 23, 101
Hayes 24, 101
Head 28, 101
Healey 72, 74, 103
Heck van 28, 101
Heerdegen 72
Heine 1, 101
Heinrich 72, 76, 104
Heldaas 73, 103
Herberts 96, 97, 101, 102
Hill 74, 103
Hipp 74, 100
Hochmeister 74, 101
Hoffman 6, 101
Hoiseth 24, 26, 99
Hoy 97, 101
Huggler 81, 99
Hughes JD 4, 100
Hughes SPF 6, 101
Huie 6, 101
Huiskes 28, 101
Hukkanen 6, 101
Humeniuk 73, 100
Hundelshausen 74, 100
Hungerford 4, 102
Husby 24, 26, 99
Husebo 73, 74, 100
Hvid 23, 24, 26, 101, 102
Hyderally 74, 101
Hyland 74, 101

Ilstrup 4, 5, 74, 96, 99, 102
Im 3, 4, 5, 103
Indong 73, 101
Issendorff 73, 101, 104

Jacob 28, 104
Jasty 6, 97, 101
Jensen 24, 101, 102
Jin 48, 100
Johnson 72, 73, 97, 101
Johnston 96, 99, 104
Jolley 3, 5, 28, 101, 103
Jones DA 72
Jones LC 4, 102
Jones RH 74, 102
Joyce 5, 101
Judet 2, 3, 102

Kafka 26, 102
Kakkar 72, 73, 102, 104
Kälebo 73
Kallos 72, 73, 74, 76, 102, 104
Kaplan 6, 102
Kapper 22, 99
Karlström 72, 73, 103
Kärrholm 97, 102
Kavanagh 96, 102
Kay 67, 73, 97, 103, 104
Keenan 73, 102
Keller GS 72, 73, 103
Keller JC 52, 102

Kelley MA 73
Kelley SS 96, 104
Kenneth 74, 100
Kapes 74, 102
Kerschbaumer 34, 36, 99
Kiaer 3, 102
Kierulf 73, 103
King 24, 100
Kistner 72, 103
Kjaeer 72, 104
Kleinschmidt 3, 102
Knahr 28, 103
Kobayashi 4, 102
Koch 74, 104
Kolb 74, 100
Kong 72, 103
König 1, 102
Konttinen 6, 101
Korostoff 23, 104
Kössler 76, 103
Krause 67, 97, 102
Krug 67, 97, 102
Ku 22, 99
Kuczynski 74, 101
Kummer 24, 102
Kuner 72, 104

Lahirl 74, 103
Landauer 72, 74, 99
Landstrand 97, 104
Langeland 73, 74, 100
Lanyon 22, 24, 26, 102, 103
Larsen 26, 101
Lassen 73, 99
Laufer 74, 101
Laurensen 73, 100
Laurin 97, 102
Lautenschlager 48, 52, 100, 102
Lawrence 73, 102, 104
Lazcano 96, 102
Learmonth 5, 100
Les AJC 46, 48, 53, 67, 97, 99, 101, 102
Lee K 6, 101
Leland 97, 104
Lettin 73, 74, 103
Levell 6, 101
Lewalle 96, 102
Lidgren 48, 97, 102, 103
Liedloff 72, 73, 102
Lindahl 86, 96, 103
Lindberg 72, 103
Lindbratt 73, 100
Linde 23, 24, 102
Linder 6, 11, 97, 102
Lindstrand 97, 102
Ling 6, 46, 48, 53, 67, 97, 99, 101, 102
Locke 28, 103
Lotke 73, 102
Louden 73, 104
Loynes 73, 101
Ludin 72, 104
Lunceford 97, 104
Lush-Ehmann 72, 73, 103

Maclouf 6, 101
Madey 96, 102
Maffei 73, 104
Mahmud 23, 101
Malchau 96, 97, 101, 102
Malcolm 6, 97, 102
Maloney W 6, 101
Maloney WJ 6, 97, 101
Marder 73, 100
Maripuu 72, 73, 103

Markolf 67, 68, 97, 99, 102
Marks 5, 104
Marti 6, 104
Martin 4, 100
Martini 23, 101
Matthews 22, 23, 26, 99, 101
Maxeiner 74, 102
Mayfield 72, 103
McCarthy 6, 101
McCollister 72, 73, 103
McCutchen 5, 99
McElhaney 24, 102
McGann 4, 5, 97, 99, 101
McGrath 74, 103
McKee 2, 4, 102
McKusick 72, 101
McMinn 6, 99
McNeise 67, 68, 97, 99
Mead 6, 99
Meier 6, 102
Mellmann 72, 73, 104
Meranze 73, 102
Merenstein 72, 102
Merkel 81, 103
Merli 73, 99
Michelinakis 74, 103
Miller EH 67, 97, 103
Miller J 67, 97, 102
Miller R 74, 101
Miller WE 72, 100
Mills 24, 104
Milne 74, 103
Mitsunaga 72
Mjöberg 97, 103, 104
Modig 72, 73, 101, 103
Mogensen 97, 103
Mohler 72, 100
Möller 48, 102
Montrey 72, 103
Moore 2, 103
Morgan 74, 103
Morley 72, 102
Morscher 72, 104
Mullen 73, 103
Müller 54, 98, 103
Murray 72, 102

Naess-Andresen 73, 103
Nairn 73, 104
Neumann 96, 103
Newens 74, 103
Newman 73, 100
Nice 74, 103
Nillius 72, 73, 100, 103
Nilsen 73, 103
Noble 86, 96, 103
Nordgren 73, 101
Nylander 73, 103

Oh 68, 97, 103
Ohnsorge 73, 103
Older 3, 4, 5, 79, 83, 86, 96, 103
Olejniczak 96, 102
Olerud 73, 101
Olsen 73, 99
Olsson 97, 103
Orsini 73, 103

Paes 72, 102
Palevsky 73, 102
Panjabi 73, 100
Patterson 72, 74, 103
Paul 24, 103
Pauwels 24, 26, 103
Peebles 74, 103

Author Index

Pellegrini jr 72, 73, 103
Perren 24, 30, 103
Phillips 73, 74, 103
Pinto 6, 99
Pitto 76, 98, 99, 103
Poisel 34, 36, 99
Polak 6, 101
Pongsoipetch 23, 102
Powell 74, 103
Pretschner 72, 73, 104
Pynsent 6, 99

Radin 24, 103
Rahn 30, 103
Raugstad 73, 74, 100
Reichelt 28, 100
Richards 73, 100
Ringsdorf 72, 104
Ritter G 73, 101, 103, 104
Ritter MA 28
Robbins 74, 101
Rosberg 72, 73, 100
Rosborough 74, 101
Röttger 6, 103
Rubin 22, 24, 103
Ruckelshausen 2, 103
Rudigier 73, 97, 100, 104
Rüegsegger 26, 103
Rushdied 6, 101
Russe 97, 103
Russotti 4, 5, 96, 103
Ryd 97, 103, 104

Sagar 73, 104
Sahlstedt 72, 73, 103
Sakimura 72, 100
Salvati 2, 3, 4, 5, 28, 101, 103
Salzer 28, 103
Santavirta 6, 101
Sarmiento 32, 97, 99, 101
Sasahara 73, 99
Sauer 97
Sauri Arce 96, 102
Schatzker 28, 32, 96, 99, 101
Schemitsch 73, 100
Schlag 72, 103, 104
Schliep 72, 104
Schmidt 78, 104
Schött 73, 99
Schreiber 28, 104
Schulitz 74, 104
Schulte 96, 104
Schurmann 6, 101
Scott 23, 104
Seelig 72, 104
Seidenstein 4, 5, 101
Selvik 97, 99, 102, 103, 104
Serot 67, 97, 103
Sevitt 72, 74, 104
Shao 97, 104
Sharrock 72, 74, 103
Sherman 67, 97, 104
Sibley 6, 101
Sidney 96, 104
Siebler 72, 104
Simpson 74, 103
Slooff 3, 7, 28, 101, 104
Smith RE 4, 104
Smith TC 74, 100
Smith-Petersen 2, 104
Snorrason 97, 102
Soltesz 52, 104
Song 6, 101
Sonstegard 22, 26, 101
Soondergaard 26, 101

Sörenson 96, 103
Stadeager 72, 104
Stamatakis 73, 104
Stanley 22, 99
Stärk 28, 103
Stauffer 4, 5, 96, 102, 103, 104
Steinberg 73, 102
Stören 73, 103
Strafford 23, 99
Strand 73, 74, 100
Strauss 72
Strens 28, 101
Stride 74, 103
Strömberg 96, 101
Sullivan 67, 97, 99, 104
Summer-Smith 32, 96, 101
Sutherland CJ 5, 104
Sutherland IC 74, 104
Sychterz 24, 104

Tanaka 28, 104
Terayama 4, 5, 102, 104
Thabe 28, 104
Thomas EM 72, 102
Thomas KA 26, 100, 101
Thomas TA 74, 104
Thompson 2, 104
Thorburn 73, 104
Tigchelaar 6, 101
Tillmann B 41, 104
Tillmann K 28, 104
Tjörnstrand 97
Tolkoff 24, 103
Tomford 68, 73, 97, 101, 103
Torholm 73, 100
Trentz 72, 73, 104
Tronzo 73, 74, 104
Tscherne 72, 73, 104
Tullos 86, 96
Turner CH 24, 104
Turner RJ 4, 104
Tzitzikalakis 3, 4, 5, 100

Ulrich 72, 76, 100, 104
Underwood 74, 102

Vakili 3, 5, 103
Vallance 73, 104
Van Der Vis 6, 104
Van Noorden 6, 104
Vangala 67, 97, 101
Volz 74, 103
Von Issendorff 73
Von Langenbeck 1

Waddell 67, 73, 97, 103, 104
Wagner 28, 104
Walker 24, 104
Waltman 72, 101
Ward 73, 102
Waring 2, 99
Waterhouse 74, 104
Watson-Farrar 2, 4, 102
Weidenreich 25, 104
Weinstein 97, 104
Weitz 73, 99
Wells 73, 100
Wenda 73, 104
Westermann 72, 73, 104
Wilde 5
Wilke 28, 100
Wille-Jörgensen 72, 104
Willenegger 97, 100
Williams 4, 5, 101
Willner 97, 103

Wilson DL 22, 26, 101
Wilson PD jun. 2, 3, 4, 5, 103
Winter-Christensen 72, 104
Wixon 48, 100
Woolson 6, 101
Wörsdörfer 72, 76, 104
Wrighton 5, 48, 102
Wroblewski 3, 4, 5, 79, 96, 104

Wyche 73, 74, 104

Yew 86, 96, 103

Zichner 74, 104
Zimmermann 73, 99
Zippel 72

Acknowledgements

The authors wish to acknowledge the great support received by Springer-Verlag for the venture of assembling this manual. In particular, we wish to thank the editor Mrs. Gabriele Schröder and the technical coordinator Mrs. Ute Pfaff for their marvellous attention to this project. Furthermore, we wish to thank Mr. Reinhold Henkel for his expert anatomical drawings and Mr. Joachim Schmidt for the excellent layout.

We are indebted to all collaborators of the ZOW who contributed to the research and the publication.

Printing and binding: Druckerei Triltsch, Würzburg